WE THE PATIENTS

How America's Health Care System Was Hijacked and What We Must Do to Reclaim the Soul of Medicine

Copyright © 2009 Sam JW Romeo, MD, MBA, with Steve Fox
All rights reserved.

ISBN: 1-4392-5014-6
EAN13: 9781439250143

Visit www.booksurge.com to order additional copies.

WE THE PATIENTS

How America's Health Care System Was Hijacked and What We Must Do to Reclaim the Soul of Medicine

Sam JW Romeo, MD, MBA, with **Steve Fox**

FORWARD

This book examines the deterioration of America's health care system, identifies the primary causes and provides recommendations on how to remedy matters. My observations are not theoretical – they arise from more than 40 years on the frontlines of health care. I have been an ER physician, a family physician seeing 25 to 35 patients a day and delivering 100-plus babies and performing 60-plus major surgeries a year, head of a multi-specialty medical group practice, and operator of a network of clinics for the rural poor in Idaho. I have treated indigent patients in storefront ghetto clinics, developed emergency and ambulatory care networks, and run small HMOs in several states. I helped create a widely-praised, employer-funded health delivery plan for Fortune 1000 member Johnson Controls Inc. and later, as Senior Associate Dean of the University of Southern California School of Medicine, founded what became the nation's first fully accredited Independent Physicians Association, University Affiliates IPA.

Throughout my career, improving and ensuring the quality of health care has been a foremost concern of mine, and I have lectured and taught widely on the subject. I am a past President of the Accreditation Association for Ambulatory Health Care, Inc., and in 1998 I was honored to be named Physician Executive of the Year by the American College of Medical Practice Executives. I have dedicated my life to providing medical care to individuals and to working to improve America's health care institutions.

I mention all this to make you aware that although my primary orientation is that of a family physician, I have seen health care from all angles. Although I'm still active in health care on a daily basis, I'm not pushing any group's agenda, running for any office, or looking for any favors. What I have to say is going to irritate people at high levels, which is probably good for them, and the solutions I propose are going to require each of us to think and behave in different ways.

Unhappily, my career coincides with a period in which many Americans went from being generally satisfied with their health care experiences to being outraged by them. I have been buffeted, both personally and professionally, by the perversities of our health care system and I have encountered both frustration and success in my attempts to improve things. However, I continue to believe that an equitable, effective and compassionate health care system is both possible and imperative.

This is a real-world book, not an academic treatise. Although I have written dozens of articles for various medical publications, I have in this book avoided salting my observations with studies and footnotes, choosing instead to illustrate my points primarily with real-life examples. This reflects my strong belief that while our health care system has become horribly complex, the forces that damaged it are common – greed, self-centeredness, arrogance, and ignorance are some that come to mind.

Like all authors, my values and beliefs are on display here, so I think it's appropriate that you ask – and that I answer – the question of why you should listen to me on this subject. In my view, a full answer requires telling you more about my background – not out of ego on my part, I hope – but so that you will have a perspective from which to judge the observations I'm going to make. I am beholden to no one except my maker, and I'm not carrying water for any politician or special interest group. What I say here reflects what I've seen and experienced personally, not what anyone wants me to say. And so you'll understand where I'm coming from, let me tell you, literally, where I came from.

I was born in 1940 in my grandparents' home in Ely, NV, a common occurrence at that time in the rural high desert of northeastern Nevada. My parents were first-generation Americans born and raised in the same town. My family was dirt-poor, although we didn't think of ourselves that way. My father, who worked as a welder, borrowed $200 from a local banker the year I was born and paid $5 an acre for 40 sagebrush-studded acres outside of town. It ultimately became the Romeo Ranch, but it wasn't much to begin with.

My father fenced and cleared the land, digging a well six feet in diameter and twenty feet deep with a pick and shovel. Within a year he had planted his first crop and purchased a chicken coop which he moved onto the ranch and rebuilt to become our family home. We slowly built or acquired farm machinery and began to raise horses, cows and alfalfa, eventually leasing an adjoining 160-acre property where we moved and expanded our original home. My brother and I worked throughout our youths as farmhands.

We acquired our first electric generator when I was about 12. Soon after that, a propane furnace replaced the wood fireplace and kitchen stove as interior heat. We still had no inside plumbing. When I was 14, we dug another well and built a 25-foot wood frame structure and mounted atop it a 2,000-gallon water tank, insulating the tank from the 30-below winter cold with wool shorn from our sheep. A hand-built windmill pumped water into a hand-built plumbing system that piped water through coils in the kitchen wood stove and into a 50-gallon tank that served as a hot water reservoir. We created a bathroom by partitioning off a portion of the back porch and were finally able to take hot showers inside the house. Four years later, when I left for college, it was only the third time I had ever traveled further away from home than you could ride on horseback in one day.

How did someone with this kind of background become a physician? My mother had some training as a nurse, and the town's veterinarian was a close family friend before he died, leaving his veterinary books to my father. My father absorbed the books and became the resident veterinarian for ranchers within 75 miles of our ranch. I enjoyed accompanying him on his "consultations" and a seed was planted. Also, my brother was a far better horseman than I, so he became the cowboy and I became the "doctor." While he was herding, roping and holding the calf, I would dehorn, wattle, vaccinate, castrate, and brand it. My father was forever present, helping and teaching. Graduating from animals to humans seemed a natural progression, and a physician was the only thing I ever wanted to be.

I received my B.S. degree from St. Mary's College in Northern California and my M.D. degree from Saint Louis University's School of Medicine. My vision then of being a doctor was to be like those few physicians who provided health care in our tiny community – all general practitioners. In fact, I was in med school before I ever fully recognized that there were several different types of physicians. How naïve I was and how much I had to learn! But the more I did learn about medicine and its various specialties, the more committed I became to being a family doctor and to treating people who had inadequate health care services. I have spent much of my medical career fulfilling that commitment.

I met my wife Patty when I was a sophomore in college, and my world changed. Things that had been impossible became possible. Rough-edged off the ranch and plagued with a reading disability, I had always struggled as a student. After meeting her, I made the honor roll. My dream of becoming a physician, derided by my high school counselors, now seemed within reach. I was enormously fortunate – Patty and I filled each other's gaps and became as one in pursuing our goals of having a family and making it through med school.

Achieving the first goal was pretty easy. Patty and I had five children in four and a half years (she won the fertility award in our class). With all the obligations that this presented, I grabbed the opportunity to join the Navy in my junior year of med school and get a regular paycheck. We needed that paycheck badly – I was simultaneously a med student and a Food Stamp recipient, standing in line with my white coat and white face setting me very much apart from the others around me. When I completed school, I was selected for one of the four Family Medicine seats available each year in all the U.S. Armed Forces. I did my internship in the Navy at Camp Pendleton Marine Corp Base in California and my residency in Jacksonville, FL. My first duty station was Port Hueneme, CA, where we had our sixth and final child. Five of our children have become physicians and the sixth is a Licensed Clinical Social Worker. My family is by far my most important achievement.

My wife has been my partner throughout everything, including this book, and so I thought it was appropriate that she have the opportunity to make some observations of her own about the kind of man I am. What follows are her comments, unedited and uncensored by me:

"My husband truly loves the profession of medicine, so he naturally wants to try to save what he believes is being destroyed. I think one of his motivations for writing this book is that he sees medicine as a noble profession that is being torn apart by bureaucrats. Throughout his life, he has always looked at ways to fix things or make things better. There is a purity to his way of thinking that is sometimes unrealistic and has made our lives challenging at times. He genuinely tries to do what is good for people as a whole rather than what is good for him as an individual. He is motivated by his principles and has never let someone else's opinion of him rule him.

"There have been times when his Italian passion was misunderstood for anger. Could he have said things in a gentler way? Probably. But that wouldn't have been the man of commitment that I married years ago. He has never been afraid to question authority or the status quo, especially when the "party line" threatens people or his principles.

"Sam has an unbelievable capacity to love and the faith that God will never send more than we can handle. His philosophy is that if a person is doing the right action for the right reason, things will work out. My husband has always walked the walk. He went into medicine, he went into medical management, and he wrote this book, all out of his love for taking *care of people. For Sam, it has never been about the money or about his career or about fame. All through our nearly 50 years of being together, his commitment to me and all his family, which now includes our 21 grandchildren, has been limitless."*

She's right, as usual, and I plead guilty as charged. I wrote this book because I'm certain we can and should have a better health care system than we do now, because I think I know where we went wrong, and because I believe I see what we need to do to fix things. My goal is to punch through all the misconceptions and self-serving observations that surround our current dialogue on health care and bring some reality to the discussion. If I can contribute to repairing and reforming our health care system, I will be gratified.

Thank you for buying my book. If you have a comment on what I have to say, I'd like to hear it. My email address is drromeo@wethepatients.org.

Sam JW Romeo, MD, MBA
Turlock, CA

WE THE PATIENTS

*How America's Health Care System Was Hijacked
And What We Must Do to Reclaim the Soul of Medicine*

TABLE OF CONTENTS

Chapter One
America's Health Care Crisis 1

Chapter Two
A System We Never Planned 15

Chapter Three
The Doctor-Patient Relationship Is in Critical Condition . . . 41

Chapter Four
How Our Profit-Driven Health Care System Corrupts
Medical Decision-Making 55

Chapter Five
How Health Care Came to Focus on Diseases
Rather Than Patients. 73

Chapter Six
How the House of Medicine Fragmented And
What That Means to Patients. 87

Chapter Seven
An Overdose of Greed.............................101

Chapter Eight
Damaged in Medical School 129

Chapter Nine
Why We Have to Ration Health Care And
How to Do It Compassionately 147

Chapter Ten
Re-imagining Health Care..........................161

Chapter Eleven
What Each of Us Can and Must Do To Reclaim Control
of Our Health and Health Care System 183

Chapter Twelve
The Future of American Health Care 197

Chapter One

AMERICA'S HEALTH CARE CRISIS

Why Only We the Patients Offer Real Hope for a Solution

One of the few positive things you can say about America's health care crisis is that very few people are in denial about it anymore. We know things are a mess, because of what happens to us personally when we need medical care, because of what it costs, and because of what we see in the media. We know that the health care crisis is a complex and multifaceted issue, with convenient scapegoats often substituting for impartial inquiry and thoughtful dialogue about what is really wrong. We know that our health care "system" is badly broken. And deep down, whatever our level of knowledge about American health care, we know that it shouldn't and doesn't have to be this way.

I put quotes around "system" because what we have today isn't a system at all. Modern American health care is more akin to a jungle, where patients often feel like prey and many providers and payers behave like predators. The strong are surviving, but many of us are deeply – and justifiably – afraid of what would happen if we or someone we love faced a serious health issue. How did things reach this point, and what can we do about it?

Like most difficult problems, America's health care crisis is multi-determined. There is no single cause, no handy villain to blame, and no quick solution. In fact, many of the thorniest issues took root in the best of intentions, and some of the most pernicious problems are unexpected by-products of previous efforts to improve the system. A lot of very smart people have attempted to "fix" our health care system. That they have failed is testament to the challenges we face.

Unlike almost all other industrialized countries, America never created a comprehensive national mechanism for delivering health care to those who live here. Instead, we let health care develop within the framework of the profit-centered free enterprise system, enacted enormously expensive government programs aimed at helping specific groups, grafted other programs onto those, stood by while crafty entrepreneurs reached into our collective pockets, then reacted with repair efforts which in turn attracted more money-hungry parasites.

What we have today wasn't planned. It metastasized, fed by an ever-increasing share of our Gross Domestic Product. What's worse, we've now reached a point where what is rightfully called the medical-industrial complex is so entrenched, so rich, and so powerful that meaningful health care reform isn't going to originate in Washington.

In other words, we're not going to get a "top-down" solution. Our leaders, and in particular our legislators, have been thoroughly co-opted and corrupted by the massive amounts of money flowing from the health care industry to those who influence and regulate it. And it goes further than Washington. Medical schools, regulatory agencies, professional societies, and other societal institutions that should be looking out for us are instead looking out for themselves, and doing quite nicely, thank you. The very institutions that should be protecting us have become revolving-door training grounds for those who learn how to game the system and then sell that knowledge to the highest bidder.

Our alleged leaders and institutions can get away with this partially because we don't really know how they feel about health care. Is it a right or a privilege? Should some basic level of health care be available to anyone living here, citizen or not? How much of our national income should be spent on health care? Accepting the reality that we can't provide everyone with all the medical care they might want, how should we allocate our finite health care resources? How big a role should government play in health care? How big a role should private enterprise play?

Because we've never really dealt with these and other fundamental questions, what we now have isn't working for anyone. Even being really rich or having great insurance doesn't guarantee that you'll receive timely treatment in an emergency room – because it's almost certain to be crammed with folks who go there for basic care because they can't afford health insurance.

America's current health care "model" – quotes again, because what we have is an accident, not a plan – is oriented almost entirely toward providing high-cost treatment to people with chronic conditions. We do this episodically, not in any methodical way. We are disease-oriented and reactive – we wait until people have serious health issues and then throw money at their problems. What this means from a financial standpoint is that about 75% of our health care dollars go to treat chronic illnesses such as asthma, diabetes, heart disease, and others. Not all but most of these illnesses are lifestyle-related, which means they are largely preventable. In other words, the majority of the $2 trillion we spend every year on health care goes to treat diseases people didn't have to develop in the first place.

Why is this happening? As I will explain in the following chapters, there are a number of reasons, but a large part of it is that we don't personally feel the financial pain that our lifestyle decisions – and those of others – create. While almost everyone complains – and rightly so – about the high cost of health care, only 13% of the total expenditures come directly out of consumers' pockets. Because of the way our health care system evolved, there's a widespread illusion that somebody else (government, employers, insurance companies) is paying. They're not. You and I are.

If you can get to it, the overall quality of American health care is generally very good. It may no longer be the best in the world, and in some areas we are performing poorly, but any honest examination of other countries' health care systems will find significant flaws there too. What does work in another country is only somewhat relevant to our situation anyway – America is different from every other country in a variety of ways. In other words, we're also not going to find a solution to our health care crisis overseas. That's not to say that we can't learn from the health care systems of other nations, but the idea that we can somehow transplant what works in another country into ours is simplistic at best.

Where we as a nation have fallen down badly is the method by which we organize, deliver and finance health care. In part, this reflects Americans' inherent distrust of centralized systems for handling societal needs as well as our reluctance to place restraints on the capitalist economic model to which we are accustomed. Our history as a people is one of enduring difficulties until they reach a critical point, then responding with massive government programs intended to obliterate the problem. In the case of health care, that attitude has helped create the crisis we now face. At the same time, our other default approach – letting the parties involved slug it out in the marketplace – isn't going to cut it either. When it comes to health care, relying on market forces simply doesn't work. What we have now isn't a free market, it's a free-for-all.

Although it is endlessly peddled by those who profit from it, the concept that health care is a free market is ludicrous on its face. It's ludicrous simply because there is not free choice on the part of consumers. People don't choose to develop Alzheimer's or break an arm anymore than they choose whether or not to eat. There are certain human needs that are not discretionary, and a basic level of health care is one of them.

Taking a broader economic view for just a moment, what have so-called free markets done for us? Many of America's vital industries – finance, housing, and manufacturing among them – are in shambles. We are beholden to other countries for the oil our economy must have to function. We owe other nations more than we can possibly repay and our economy has been teetering on the brink of another Depression. A primary cause of all this is the unchecked greed of those who hide behind the smokescreen of free markets to enrich themselves. In terms of health care, free markets enable the CEOs of health care companies to take home millions while senior citizens have to choose between eating or filling their prescriptions. There is something terribly wrong with this picture.

At the same time, the "solution" being pushed by those on the other end of the political spectrum – in this case, single-payer or government-run health care – also doesn't work. Without getting into a long discussion on this issue, think of it this way: If you like dealing with the DMV, you'll love single-payer health care.

As I will show in the following chapters, our current health care crisis began with the well-intentioned government programs known as Medicare and Medicaid. These programs established a playing field on which "market forces" created the dysfunctional spectacle of medical costs driving millions of folks into bankruptcy while making a few rich beyond belief.

There are zealots on both side of this issue. Those who believe in single-payer (government) health care go to great lengths to label their opponents as rapacious capitalists. Free market proponents contend that single-payer advocates are socialists. Neither charge is true, and all the inflammatory rhetoric obscures the most important point: While we have to reform our health care system, we have to start from where we are now. We need both the oversight function of government and the innovation and efficiency of capitalism in our health care system.

There are essentially three parties in the health care equation – payers, patients and providers. Each party has its own set of needs and wants, which sometimes conflict and sometimes coincide with those of the others. What is cost for one party is income for another. There's no way around that inherent conflict – the only relevant question is how we deal with it. Unfortunately, the parties have become combatants rather than collaborators, adversaries instead of allies. This must change if we are to find a rational method for delivering health care.

There are some positive factors underlying the current situation. For one thing, what we're spending on health care right now is sufficient to fund an equitable system that provides good basic health care to all those who live here. That doesn't mean everyone gets everything they want – we're going to have to face up to the reality that health care has to be rationed. But there's plenty of money – we just don't distribute it intelligently.

Another positive factor is the one I mentioned at the beginning. We know – individually and as a nation – that our health care system has to change. No one can reasonably contend that it's working. That doesn't mean that meaningful reform won't be enormously difficult, nor that well-heeled special interests won't fight fiercely to protect their positions at the trough, but I believe the tide has truly turned against all those who get rich on the suffering of others.

Although they have each played a part, the root cause of our health care crisis is not corrupt insurance companies, drug firms, hospital chains and HMOs. It's also not greedy doctors, illegal aliens helping themselves to our hospitals, wasteful government programs or bungling bureaucrats. American health care has been damaged by all of these things, but they have been able to hurt us primarily because we have never reached a consensus within our society as to what health care should be. We have no common ground or overarching set of principles or foundational starting point for health care, and we therefore don't really know what we want or where we're going. In that kind of unstructured, valueless environment – the jungle I mentioned earlier – our basest instincts take over.

Our health care crisis is generally portrayed as something that's overwhelmingly complicated, requiring endless numbers of studies and dozens of government programs to even begin to make a difference. And while there are plenty of smart, self-interested folks spinning this story, it simply isn't true. While genetics and luck play significant roles, most chronic diseases are rooted in lifestyle choices. In other words, we each have enormous influence over our personal health. As to our health care system, it is indeed complex. But that's not the whole story. Because this complexity works to their financial advantage, many health care industry executives and other alleged experts scoff at the idea that adopting some fairly simple principles would resolve most of our system's problems.

The reality is that our health care system is complex because we have made it so, not because it is that way inherently. Medicine itself is complex, and getting more so every day as we find new ways to diagnose and treat. But what ails our financing and delivery systems is fairly straightforward. At all levels – individual patient, family, employer, provider, insurer, health care corporation, government, etc. – we're not taking responsibility for our actions and we're not holding others accountable for theirs. Our core problem is not organizational, it's ethical. Ultimately, this is a question of values.

Each of us can exert significant influence on our individual health and on our health care system. Patients who damage their individual health and then expect providers to do whatever it takes to deal with the consequences are placing a burden on everyone else. Providers – individual and corporate – who try to make health care a road to riches are exploiting their fellow man, pure and simple. Payers who manipulate the intricacies of our health care system to maximize their profits and pump up their stock prices are doing the same. These are ethical issues.

If we are to structure a system that puts patients before profits while also recognizing the role of legitimate capitalism (which is not what we have now) in health care, we're going to have to decide what our values are in this important area. This requires that we each reflect on what we believe, debate our beliefs with others and arrive at some consensus that can be translated into specifics. Only then can we structure a new model that respects and meets the needs of patients, providers and payers within a realistic understanding of our society's finite resources.

As members of American society, you and I have a basic level of financial responsibility to each other when it comes to health care. This is the underlying principle of insurance – spread the financial burden among many and it becomes tolerable for each person. What we have been reluctant to get out in the open is that when it comes to health care, my behavior affects you financially – and vice versa. I believe one of the reasons for this is that most people don't fully realize that they're paying for their own health care, as well as the health care of others.

Because of the way our system evolved, with health care insurance being primarily employer-based and government programs picking up much of the cost for millions of the elderly and poor, the connection between individual behavior and collective cost is not readily apparent. It's there, however, and we need to talk about it, if for no other reason than we've run out of money. Health care expenditures now account for 17% of our economy and are headed higher. Without reform and restraint, health care expenditures will crowd out other vital societal needs in the years ahead.

Our health care crisis is often framed in terms of cost, and there's no question that this is an important aspect of the overall problem. Too often, however, not enough is said about what each of us can gain by thinking about our individual health and our nation's health care system in a different way. After 40 years on the frontlines of health care, I believe that the discussion needs to move away from cost and onto benefit. In other words, let's stop trying to "scare" people into thinking and acting differently and talk specifically about what a new perspective can do for each of us and for our society as a whole.

I believe that most Americans can live longer and more satisfying lives, enjoy good health in their later years and face the inevitability of death with serenity and acceptance. These benefits are within our individual and collective grasp, right here, right now. They are affordable and achievable if we reject certain things that we have been conditioned to believe and instead live in ways that respect our own individual health and the fact that our personal choices affect society as a whole.

Although we've come to regard it as something we turn to only when we're sick, health care can and should be a great ally in our lives. The tools we need to enjoy healthier lives are here now, and more are on the way. We need only to pick them up and use them. Many people already have – the anecdotal evidence is all around us in the form of people who are living healthy, productive, joyous lives well into their older years.

In general terms, and I will have more to say about this later, this means that we need to teach and practice wellness and prevention. We need to be accountable – to ourselves, to those we love, and to our society as a whole – for the lifestyle choices we make every day. We need to call out and confront those who are exploiting patients for the sake of profits. And we need to recognize the reality that our health care resources are finite, that not everyone can have all the health care they believe they should have.

While this next point may sound cold-hearted, it's simply realistic. Fundamental reform of our health care system means focusing not on those who are already ill but on those who are not. The way we operate now – wait until people get sick, often because of their own lifestyle choices, and then spend huge sums of money on their problems – means that about 10% of our population drives roughly 70% of our healthcare expenditures and policy priorities. The tail is wagging the dog. We can't fix things by focusing on the symptom – we have to work on the cause. That doesn't mean abandoning those who are already ill – we have an obligation to care for them – but it does mean recognizing that we've been focusing on the wrong thing.

In broad terms, we need a greatly increased emphasis on long-term initiatives in the areas of education, wellness and prevention. This should begin in the family home and continue in what is now being called the medical home, which I will discuss in more detail. Some of the key principles of the medical home include the following:

- Health care is personal and rests on a collaborative relationship between the patient and a primary care physician.
- The patient's relationship with the primary care physician should provide continuity, availability, and coordination of care.
- That relationship should be comprehensive, encompassing well care, preventive care, acute and chronic sick care, and end-of-life care.
- The medical home should be accessible 24/7 and contain a complete health care record for every patient.
- The medical home should provide quality health care that is evidence-based and physician-directed.

For our system as a whole, our most urgent priorities include:

- Producing more primary care physicians and fewer specialists.
- Keeping healthy people healthy through wellness and prevention incentives.
- Providing quick, rational, coordinated, complete and evidence-based care to the sick.
- Emphasizing rehabilitation with incentives that reward productive lifestyles.
- Emphasizing individual and family responsibility for our own health.
- Measuring accountability first at the patient level, not at the population level.

I mentioned earlier that we are not going to get a "top-down" solution and that we can't import a cure for our health care problems. The truth is that we each have to look in the mirror. We are all consumers of health care. We all pay for the health care of ourselves and others. Although it may not seem like it, this commonality is our greatest resource in terms of changing the system. We are all in this boat, and it is sinking. Our health care system is collapsing.

As I will show, the executives of publicly-held health care companies – the big pharmaceutical firms, the hospital chains, the medical device manufacturers, the insurance companies – are worrying about their stock options, not about you and me. Our politicians have been co-opted, as have our med school professors and deans. These folks essentially believe that they can spend their way out of their personal health care problems and they are focused on amassing enough wealth to do that. There are exceptions, yes, but in the chapters that follow I will demonstrate that what I have just described is much more pervasive than I think you realize. The entrenched interests – and they are very powerful – are not going to help us.

If that's the case, to whom do we turn? There's really only one answer, which is why I chose it as the title of this book: We the Patients. We are all patients – consumers of health care if you will. This is the single role that binds us all together. If we want to change the system, we're it, and the time is right now.

We are currently experiencing what amounts to a giant wake-up call in this country. Our societal institutions have failed us, pure and simple, and we need to rethink them from top to bottom. At the individual level, personal responsibility has taken a back seat to immediate gratification, with devastating consequences. Nothing is going to really change until each of us decides that we've had enough and that we're not going to take it anymore. Real and lasting change is only going to occur as the result of a grassroots movement that pushes ethics and values up into our health care system.

The good news is that we each have more power than we believe. This is true in part because we fund the medical-industrial complex – through our taxes, the insurance premiums we pay and allow to be deducted from our paychecks, the checks we write for the co-pays, and all the other ways we spend our health care dollars. It's true also because millions of us are also shareholders in health care companies – through the stocks and mutual funds that we hold as individuals and in our company and union and personal pension plans. This is our money, and we have a say in how and where it's invested.

If all this sounds pessimistic and "negative," rest assured that it is not. In fact, I am more optimistic than ever about our chances of achieving real reform.

People are fed up and ready for change. But just as a doctor must identify an illness in order to treat it, we cannot address the problems in our health care system unless we understand what they really are and where they originated.

Let's look at how we got into this mess.

Chapter Two

A SYSTEM WE NEVER PLANNED

How Good Intentions and Bad Actors Got Us into This Mess

Every life has milestones, and one of my biggest occurred on June 4, 1966 when I graduated from Saint Louis University's School of Medicine at the age of 25. In the audience were my parents, Ab and Phyllis; my wife Patty, and our five children. More than 20 years later, as Dean of Clinical Affairs at that same medical school, I would drape cassocks over the shoulders of my sons Anthony, Joseph and Michael to signify that they too had become physicians. Still later, as Senior Associate Dean of the Medical College of Wisconsin School of Medicine, I would do the same thing when my daughter Lisa graduated. Also at Wisconsin, I looked on with great pride as another daughter, Gina, received her Masters degree. She is now a Licensed Clinical Social Worker. My youngest son, Samuel, graduated from the University of Southern California School of Medicine, where I was Senior Associate Dean, and I watched him get his diploma too.

Everything seemed possible on that marvelous June day. Patty and I had surmounted not only the usual challenges of med school but the additional difficulties of being poor and of having a big family at a young age. Our hands and hearts were full to overflowing. Perhaps in part because of this, I didn't recognize the fundamental changes that began that same year to erode the landscape of American medicine. More than 40 years later, and despite watching it occur in front of me, I still find it astonishing that we have devolved so rapidly from a health care system that generally served us well to one that is actually harming our collective health.

To see how this happened, I'm going to ask you to take a small dose of history. This won't hurt (I promise). A little history lesson is important because it explains how we came to a state where people live in fear of being bankrupted by illness, stay at jobs they despise so they won't lose their health coverage, have to choose between eating and buying their medications, and don't trust the doctors who treat them. This is nothing short of insane, and if we'd known this was where we'd wind up, we never would have started down the path I'm about to describe. Please stay with me, and when we finish you'll know how we got into this mess.

• • •

Although the U.S. is today the only major industrial country that doesn't have universal health care coverage, efforts to enact some kind of national health care program for Americans date back almost 100 years. Theodore Roosevelt proposed national health insurance in his unsuccessful 1912 Presidential campaign. President Harry Truman probably came closest, shortly after World War II, but was defeated by a coalition of forces led by the American Medical Association (AMA), which invoked the specter of "socialized medicine" to defeat what it viewed as a threat to doctors' livelihoods and patient care. For reasons I will discuss shortly, many people came to be covered by job-based private health insurance in the 1940s and 1950s, but as the 1960s began and President John F. Kennedy was elected, one group was woefully and obviously under-insured – the elderly.

What Kennedy termed "Medicare" was a central part of his domestic agenda, but the young President was stymied by AMA-led opposition and it was master politician Lyndon Johnson who was able to get Medicare passed into law as President in 1965. His hand strengthened by a substantial Democratic majority in Congress and grassroots support for his dead predecessor's initiatives, Johnson essentially co-opted opponents of the plan by giving them what they wanted. As originally enacted, Medicare would pay doctors their "usual and customary" fees, and hospitals would be compensated *based on what it cost them* to provide the specified services (*emphasis mine*). After a fierce internal debate, the AMA reluctantly went along with the new program.

What Johnson signed into law, during a celebratory ceremony at aging former President Truman's Missouri home, had three key components: 1) compulsory hospital insurance for those over 65 (Medicare Part A), 2) voluntary insurance subsidized by the government that paid doctor bills for those over 65 (Medicare Part B), and 3) federal financial assistance to state governments intended to help them provide health care to the poor (what is now Medicaid). Interestingly, Medicaid was added almost as an afterthought to the Medicare legislation and became law with relatively little debate.

Not long after winning the Medicare fight, President Johnson, alarmed by a perceived "doctor shortage," pushed through federal programs which significantly increased funding for medical students. The health care environment had thus been altered in two fundamental ways – the government was pouring money into the system, and more and more doctors were graduating and setting up shop.

If you didn't live through those years, it's difficult to appreciate fully the "no limits" mentality that prevailed during the 1960s. Johnson envisioned and attempted to create what he saw as "The Great Society" built on unrestrained federal spending and the notion that people were entitled to have the government protect them from the vicissitudes of life. Young people spurned their elders' values for an anything-goes culture whose credo, courtesy of a drug-addled Timothy Leary, was "turn on, tune in and drop out." The stock market took off, as did inflation. As the decade closed, the U.S. cemented its spot as the most powerful nation in the world by fulfilling President Kennedy's goal of putting a man on the moon. No one seemed very concerned about what all this was going to cost, and very few paid attention to the fact that personal responsibility was no longer "in". The "Me Generation" reigned supreme, with consequences we never imagined.

I mentioned earlier that private, job-based health insurance had become the primary payment mechanism for those under 65. What is generally accepted as the first private insurance plan to cover patients' hospital expenses was created in 1929 at Baylor University Hospital in Dallas, TX by an enterprising hospital administrator who offered teachers in the city's public schools this deal: Provided that 75% of the school system's teachers enrolled, those who paid 50 cents a month into a "sick benefit fund" were guaranteed up to 20 days of hospital care each year. As you might imagine, the program was a hit.

By collecting a modest amount of money every month from a large pool of individuals, only a few of whom would need care at any given time, Baylor University Hospital was applying the most basic principle of insurance – spread the risk. Other hospitals in Texas and in other states got into the act, eventually banding together to offer those who bought insurance the option of being treated at different facilities. A few years later, a Minnesota hospital insurance plan began using a blue cross in its advertising and an icon was born.

It's important to note that these early Blue Cross plans, which were non-profits, also agreed, as Medicare had, to reimburse hospitals based on their costs. However, there was no generally accepted definition of "cost." In other words, a procedure cost what the providing hospital said it cost. Remember that.

Because the financial success of these plans depended on enrolling large numbers of people, the early Blue Cross programs focused their marketing efforts primarily on self-selected groups, sometimes fraternal organizations like the Elks but more often the employees of large companies. This seemed like "win-win" – employees knew they were covered and hospitals, which had been writing off a lot of charity care, knew they would get paid. Employers liked the idea too, since it promised a healthier and more loyal workforce, and would like it even more when the IRS ruled that companies could take a tax deduction for the costs of providing employee health insurance. As the 1930s came to a close, the Blue Cross model was firmly established, and its offshoot, Blue Shield, also had been established (in 1939) to apply the same principles to the coverage of doctors' bills. Although cautious at first, the AMA ultimately endorsed the Blue Shield concept, in large part because the plan agreed to pay any qualified provider a patient chose, with physicians remaining free to set their fees according to what was "usual and customary." Once again, a given course of treatment cost what the provider said it cost, a methodology that would prove ruinous later on.

World War II changed the employment landscape, since many of America's able-bodied men were sent overseas. Competition for workers and raw materials among employers became intense, creating inflationary pressures on wages and prices that in turn generated government controls on both. However, in 1942 the Wage Labor Board ruled that while companies could not offer higher wages to attract employees, they could increase fringe benefits, i.e. health insurance. This ruling, coupled with the aforementioned IRS decision that companies could deduct the cost of providing health care, put American employers in a very powerful position vis-a-vis their workers. Firms that manufactured ball bearings or made movies were now deciding what kind of health care a pregnant woman should receive.

Think about that for a moment – your employer is deciding what your health insurance should cover and what it shouldn't. Would you let your employer decide what schools your kids can attend, or what car you drive, or what kind of food you eat? Not likely. Employer-controlled health coverage didn't happen in other countries, and it didn't happen here through any planned process or accompanied by any debate or discussion. It's taken for granted today, but job-based health coverage was essentially an accident, a byproduct of wartime worker shortages and an unusually generous IRS.

I mentioned earlier that we never would have taken this path if we knew where it led. But at the time, little if any thought was given to the ramifications of this new way of providing health coverage. Workers generally viewed it as a great perk, and enrollment in employer-paid hospital plans soared. Over time, employees came to regard health insurance as something that came with the job. Although they were now receiving what became a significant part of their compensation as a benefit – i.e., in lieu of higher take-home pay – few employees questioned the arrangement. A different attitude toward health insurance evolved. It became an entitlement, something to be used without much thought as to the financial consequences for the payer and for the system as a whole.

The enormous growth in employer-based health insurance also sparked the interest of insurance companies who sold life, property and other lines of insurance, and they later entered the health care market and began to compete with the Blues. Private insurers had been wary of health insurance, fearing that they could not price it accurately and would wind up on the hook for costly claims. However, private insurers came to like employer-based health insurance because they got access to a relatively healthy pool of individuals who were less likely to file claims (since those who were too old or too sick to work were by definition not covered), and because employers handled many of the administrative details, including deducting the premiums from employees' paychecks.

The trend towards employer-provided health coverage gained even more strength during the 1950s, with labor unions pushing for more comprehensive health benefits at contract time, a regularly-repeated phenomenon that decades later would put American automakers in the strange position of spending more on health care for every car that came off their assembly lines than they did on steel.

Make no mistake, there were still plenty of people without health care coverage during the 1960s, but the precedent of employer-provided, cost-based health insurance had been firmly established. Physicians and hospitals were still providing large amounts of uncompensated care, but the mechanisms that would put employers, insurance companies and the government squarely in the middle of American medicine had put down deep roots and could not be dislodged. Figuratively speaking, there was now another party in the examining room with the doctor and the patient – the payer – and as we were to later learn to our dismay, the payer had very different priorities than either the patient or the provider.

• • •

All this matters because it fundamentally and forever altered the relationship between patients and their doctors.

It's difficult to imagine this today, given the fractious and adversarial environment in which health care now exists, but patients and doctors once looked each other in the eye and talked not only about what had occasioned the patient's visit but also about how he or she intended to pay for the treatment the doctor was providing. Doctors knew or fairly quickly determined what an individual patient could afford to pay for a given course of treatment and tailored their charges accordingly. A simple form of what is now called "cost shifting" occurred, with doctors charging well-off patients a little more and those of modest means a little less for the same care. Wealthier folks got in to see the doctor a little sooner in the 1940s and 1950s, and might have had an extra test or two, but the overall quality of care patients received was essentially the same.

While this informal but widely understood arrangement may seem quaint or perhaps even irrelevant to today's complex and seemingly irresolvable health care issues, it actually worked pretty well. One of the main reasons, perhaps the primary reason, was the presence and force of personal responsibility, a value that has declined significantly.

We can't go back to those times, nor should we want to. Doctors can do far, far more for their patients now than they could then. Medicine has advanced since those more innocent days in ways that were unimaginable then, with individuals and our society as a whole benefiting enormously. But something also has been lost, and I believe this absence lies at the center of our current health care crisis. For a number of reasons, individual integrity and accountability are no longer core values in health care. This is true for patients, for providers and for payers.

Economists and insurance company executives have a cute term – "moral hazard" (the absence of moral values) – to describe the danger posed to an insurer by some individuals within any given group of people who have insurance. The term is thought to have originated with fire insurance companies, who recognized that a certain percentage of their customers would take out policies and subsequently set fire to their homes, but it has come to mean that one of the hazards facing insurance companies is that some of their customers aren't going to exhibit good moral behavior. They pose a "moral hazard" to insurers. These folks will hide their cars and claim they have been stolen, kill their spouses and file for death benefits, and otherwise behave in ways that are antithetical to society in general and to their insurance companies in particular.

In the case of health care insurance, particularly when it's being paid for by an employer or the government, moral hazard expresses itself in the attitude of patients who say, either openly or implicitly: "I don't care what the treatment (or operation or drug) costs. I want it, and I want it now."

On one hand, the patient's attitude is easy to understand. "What's more important than my health, or the health of my child, or mother, or father? That's what insurance is for." On the other hand, the cumulative effect of patients (and providers) saying that the cost of health care is someone else's problem is to drive that cost inexorably higher.

To be sure, there are many other factors at work in the steady rise of health care expenditures. Medicine can do much more for people today, but there are substantial costs associated with that. Inflationary pressures are certainly evident in health care, as they are in other areas of our lives. The way medicine is taught and practiced has changed significantly, and there also are considerable costs associated with that. Fear of malpractice suits have forced physicians to buy hugely expensive insurance policies, with those costs passed on, and to practice "defensive medicine" such as ordering extra tests, which also raises overall costs. And something else has changed, something fundamental. The profit motive has become an integral part of health care, pervading and corrupting every aspect of medicine.

While this may be hard to believe in today's health care environment, where doctors are routinely portrayed as opportunists and money-grubbers, I never had a single conversation with any of my medical school classmates about how much we were going to make as physicians. It wasn't part of our thought process. We believed we would make enough to take care of ourselves and our families, and that's about all we expected. I'm aware that this may sound naïve, and I don't presume to speak for all med students of that era, but that's how it was in my class. We went into medicine to help people, not to get rich. That's not the case today, and we are all suffering as a result.

• • •

The amount of money pouring into health care after the passage of Medicare caught the eyes of a lot of other people, some of them with values very different from mine. Not far away from where I was learning how to be a doctor, two young Kentucky lawyers were buying up nursing homes through a company they founded and called Extendicare. In 1968, with the stock market rising, they took the company public and shifted their focus to hospitals. Two years later, using the money raised by selling stock to investors (the initial stock zoomed from $8 a share to $80), the company had acquired 10 hospitals. In 1974, having jettisoned the nursing homes in favor of the faster-growing hospital business, the company adopted the name Humana. The name was chosen, the annual report explained: "to project more truly the philosophy of the company, to stand out distinctively and to provide an identity with non-limiting connotations." The non-limiting part must have worked. Humana would become a health care colossus, with some 80 hospitals in the U.S. and abroad.

Humana was not alone in seeing the potential in for-profit hospitals. Also in 1968, Dr. Thomas Frist Sr. and his son, Dr. Thomas Frist Jr., teamed up with an entrepreneur named Jack Massey to form Hospital Corporation of America (later shortened to HCA). The Frists, both surgeons, knew something about medicine, and Massey knew something about building companies, having previously purchased Kentucky Fried Chicken with a partner from Col. Harland Sanders and expanding it exponentially. Other for-profit, investor-owned hospital companies such as American Medical International and National Medical Enterprises (NME also was founded by lawyers) followed the lead of Humana and HCA.

The concept of publicly-held, for-profit hospital corporations, with their relentless focus on sales targets, quarterly earnings and stock options, is widely accepted today. It can therefore be difficult for people to grasp what a radical departure this idea was from the way hospitals generally operated before the late 1960s. In those days, hospitals were simply not considered businesses (the idea that a hospital would advertise was almost unthinkable). There was no such thing as the hospital "industry". Most hospitals were either government-owned, i.e., the county or city hospital; or non-profit organizations operated by a religious order or a local board of trustees. They were expected to take care of the elderly and indigent, either as government institutions serving the community or, in the case of the non-profits, to justify their tax-free status. Non-profit hospitals also frequently served as training institutions for medical students. Once again, while it wasn't a perfect system, it worked pretty well.

The creation of Medicare and Medicaid changed all this. One of the primary, if unintended, effects of the new law – and one that the lawyers who founded the for-profit hospital chains and the investors who purchased stock in them recognized quite clearly – was to relieve hospitals of the financial burden of treating many patients who could not pay, i.e., the elderly and the poor. The federal government was now paying. What had been a constant drain now converted to a revenue stream. As you will I hope remember, procedures cost what hospitals said they cost – an enviable formula that made the financial prospects for hospitals quite attractive indeed. With revenues now based on a cost-plus reimbursement formula, a hospital's profit margins were essentially guaranteed. If patient volume could be driven high enough, hefty profits were a given. Investors piled into hospital stocks, and their motivation was money, not patient care.

The action wasn't limited to hospitals. Nursing homes, firms providing home health care, labs, radiology (now called "imaging") centers, ambulatory care centers and a variety of other health care companies also went public, selling stock to investors who expected them to maximize revenues and profits. Universities began offering a new degree – Master of Hospital Administration (MHA) – which taught upcoming hospital industry executives how to navigate the complexities of Medicare/Medicaid and other payment plans. Some of these bright MHA students became very, very good at gaming the system, a skill they continue to hone to this day.

Now, one of the central realities of health care is that hospitals, clinics, labs, etc. generally get their patients through referrals from physicians. Doctors "own" their patients and send them where they choose to send them. What this means in practice is that if a hospital – or lab, or clinic, or (fill in the blank) – wants to do well financially, it had better take care of the doctors in its service area. One obvious way to do this is to cut them in on the action, i.e., offer physicians equity ownership in the facility in exchange for the ongoing referral of patients. You can probably figure out the next step, which is that a physician who owns a piece of the imaging lab down the street often somehow decides that a quite a few of his patients need X-rays.

Another way to motivate physicians to refer patients to a hospital is to help them with their expenses. Hospitals therefore began to offer physicians cut-rate rents in nearby medical office buildings. Some hospitals went further, guaranteeing private practice physicians a certain level of income in return for patient referrals, an arrangement that was particularly attractive to newly-minted doctors with substantial medical school debts, or doctors who had moved into a community and needed to build a practice from scratch. Hospital administrators and marketing directors, some using skills learned in their MHA programs, came up with all kinds of incentives.

Although these marketing practices were at first most prevalent among for-profit hospitals, that changed pretty quickly as the competition for patients intensified. Non-profits say that they are driven by their "mission," not by profits, and while that's generally true, non-profit hospitals have to pay the electric bill just like for-profits do. Non-profits use terms like "margin" or "surplus" to describe the money that's left over from revenue after all expenses are paid (what public companies would call net income or profit), and a common phrase at non-profit hospitals is: "No margin, no mission." Non-profit hospitals that wanted to survive in the new competitive environment had to adapt, and they did, by using many of the same marketing practices as the for-profits.

Most of these practices are now illegal, outlawed by the so-called "Stark laws" authored by California Congressman Pete Stark. However, any honest hospital administrator will tell you that a hospital's patient volume is still largely driven by the physicians who practice there and that successful hospitals find ways to keep those physicians happy. There was competition between hospitals, but it was primarily for the allegiance of physicians who could bring in patients, not competition on quality, and certainly not competition on price.

• • •

In many industries, and in truly free markets, competition can reasonably be expected to drive prices down. That's not true in health care, for reasons I will discuss later on. What happened in the intensifying competitive environment of the late 1960s is that health care costs rose – dramatically. Health care expenditures accounted for about 5.5% of the nation's Gross Domestic Product (GDP) in 1966, when Medicare and Medicaid took effect. Five years later, that percentage was about 7% (it's now more than 16% and headed for 20%). The costs of Medicare and Medicaid had blasted through the original projections. Government and private employers were paying more and more for health care, with no relief in sight. In just a few years, health care costs had skyrocketed – and President Richard M. Nixon was paying attention.

In 1970, Nixon set out a "new national health strategy" centered on new entities with the appealing name of "health maintenance organizations." HMOs were supposed to restrain runaway costs by providing their members with health care for a fixed monthly fee, using the clout of large memberships (generally employee groups) to negotiate financial concessions from providers (doctors, hospitals, labs, clinics, etc.). In 1973, Congress passed the HMO Act, which favored non-profit HMOs by making them eligible for various forms of federal financial assistance but also left the market open to for-profit HMOs.

The Nixon Administration and Congress had been sold on the idea of "managed care," as exemplified by HMOs, by a well-meaning physician named Paul Ellwood. The concept actually dated back to Depression-era prepaid medical group practices established by industrialist Henry Kaiser, which eventually became the Kaiser Permanente system. HMOs seemed compelling. The so-called "indemnity insurance" plans that employers had been purchasing to cover their employees' health care costs were essentially paying providers whatever they said their costs were. This kind of system obviously contained precious little incentive for the providers to limit those "costs". In fact, providers who found a way to do things more efficiently and reduce their costs also thereby reduced their reimbursement.

Ellwood, who eventually came to be dismayed at how HMOs evolved, had what at first really did seem like a better mousetrap. Managed care would do just what it sounds like – manage health care costs by reviewing and limiting the amounts and costs of health care services provided to employees covered by the now ubiquitous company-paid health insurance. Employees would be required to pay part of the premiums, often 20%, and employers would know what their overall health care costs were going to be because the HMOs were accepting a fixed amount to cover all their employees. HMOs, which were assuming the responsibility for managing health care costs and the liability if they failed, would even justify the "health maintenance" part of their names by promoting preventive health care services that would maintain the health of those they covered and therefore lead to both a healthier workforce and lower expenses. That was the theory, and until it was tested, it sounded pretty good.

Although there were variations on the core HMO concept, it essentially worked like this at inception. HMOs used their clout (they now "owned" the patients) to force primary care physicians, who became the gatekeepers to health care, to accept a fixed amount per month per patient, a payment method with the slightly chilling name of capitation. Patients (employees) had to choose a primary care physician from a group approved by their HMO. And if doctors wanted to be among that group (on the HMO's roster), they had to accept the capitation formula offered by the HMO. Patients had to get approval from their primary care physician in order to see a specialist, who also had agreed to accept the discounted fees set by the HMO for various procedures; or to enter a hospital, which also had agreed to accept what the HMO would pay. (What I have just described is the model in which physicians continue to practice independently in their own offices. There are also "Staff-model" HMOs, where the physicians are employed directly by the HMO – Group Health of Puget Sound is an example; and "Group-model" HMOs – Kaiser is an example, which contract with multi-specialty physician groups to provide both primary and specialty care.)

Initially, most HMOs were non-profits, as had once been the case with hospitals. But when federal subsidization of HMOs later withered, non-profit HMOs converted to for-profit status and today the majority of HMOs are for-profit, investor-owned corporations.

The HMO business model is fairly straightforward. Revenues come from premiums paid by the companies (usually 80%) the HMO signs up as customers, and from premiums paid by those companies' employees (usually 20%). An HMO's costs include payments to health care providers (the percentage of premiums collected actually paid out to providers is charmingly called the "medical loss ratio"), and other expenses common to investor-owned companies – salaries, bonuses, marketing, office space, general and administrative costs etc. Like all for-profit, investor-owned companies, publicly-held HMOs strive to have enough left over after all expenses are deducted from all revenues that they have turned a profit. The more profitable they are, the more successful they are in the eyes of Wall Street.

You can see where this leads. The less an HMO pays out for health care claims (HMO executives proudly tout their low medical loss ratios to Wall Street analysts), the more of those premium dollars that flow down to the bottom line. The higher the earnings per share, the better the stock generally does, which means the better the HMO executives' stock options do. The central point is that profits become more important than patients.

There was another force at work in the rise of managed care, which was the belief that the economic dynamics of the marketplace – supply and demand, open competition, etc. – were the best way to deal with complex societal issues. This reliance on so-called "free markets" and wariness of government programs ran through many of the decisions made by Nixon and Presidents Gerald Ford and George H. Bush, perhaps reaching its zenith with President Ronald Reagan, who famously declared: "Government is not a solution to our problem, government is the problem."

That there was a problem with health care spending was not open to debate. In 1980, when Reagan was elected, the U.S. was spending an estimated $257 billion on health care, up from some $73 billon in 1970. Health care spending as a percentage of GDP was closing in on 9%, and government spending on Medicare and Medicaid had soared more than five-fold over the past decade. Whatever was happening out there in the marketplace, it was not restraining health care costs.

Despite his belief in free markets and disdain for government regulations, Reagan decided to do something about an area the government could control – Medicare reimbursements. In 1983, the Reagan Administration did away with fee-for-service reimbursement (it costs what the hospital says it costs) and set forth instead a long schedule of fixed amounts that Medicare would henceforth pay for specific medical services provided in hospitals, or what were called "Diagnostic Related Groups." In other words, Medicare would reimburse providers, which it tightly defined only as hospitals, X dollars for an appendectomy, Y dollars to care for a heart attack, Z dollars for a brain tumor, and so on for a long list of widely-recognized treatments. "It-costs-what-the-provider-says-it-costs" had been replaced, at least for Medicare, by "it-costs-what-the-government-says-it-costs". DRGs, as they came to be known, would have a major impact on how medicine was paid for and practiced.

• • •

Reagan's election marked a fundamental pro-business shift in America, one that has remained intact until recently, and this shift was followed by a long and historic rise in stock values that underwrote corporate shenanigans and excesses on a previously unimaginable scale. The idea that corporate CEOs could take home annual compensation packages of $50 million, $100 million or more, unthinkable when I graduated from medical school, is common now. Remember the "Me Generation" of the 1960s? They're now firmly ensconced in executive suites and boardrooms across America.

Reflecting that pro-business shift and coinciding with Reagan's election was a major change in how new drugs would be discovered and brought to market, one that helped the pharmaceutical industry become the titan it is today. Up until that time, most research into new drugs was underwritten by the National Institute of Health (NIH) and promising discoveries were in the public domain – available to any company that wanted to take them further. The premise was that since the research was funded by taxpayers, the potentially beneficial results should be available to all. But in 1980 Congress enacted legislation that allowed universities and small companies doing NIH-funded research to patent their discoveries and then license them to the major drug companies. The NIH subsequently was allowed to enter directly into deals with Big Pharma, as the drug industry is known on Wall Street.

In other words, taxpayer-financed discoveries could become the exclusive property of big pharmaceutical corporations, which could then sell the resulting medications to consumers. (In case you weren't counting, taxpayers thus paid twice.) A few years later, in what unintentionally but ultimately became another gift to Big Pharma, Congress passed legislation that lengthened significantly the patent life for brand-name drugs. Together, these two measures meant that Big Pharma could obtain promising new drugs discovered through taxpayer-financed research from the NIH (and the universities and small companies the NIH funded), patent those drugs and keep monopoly rights to them for longer periods of time. In essence, you and I as taxpayers have partially financed the development of medications for which we are subsequently charged huge amounts of money. More on this later.

You can see the effects of these changes in today's prices for prescription drugs. What is less apparent but perhaps even more pernicious is the effect these changes have had on medical schools and teaching hospitals, where financial ties between Big Pharma and academic researchers and faculty physicians have become more and more common. These relationships have undermined the impartiality of medical research on new and existing drugs and contributed to an erosion of ethics in medical schools. Ask yourself this question: How much do I trust the findings of researchers who are investigating potential drugs that can make them personally rich if those drugs are found to be effective and become big sellers?

• • •

As the 1990s began, health care costs as a percentage of GDP had reached 12% (bear in mind that GDP itself had also increased throughout the years, so health care now accounted for a larger slice of a larger pie), and what was now being called the "medical-industrial complex" had grown wealthy indeed. With that wealth came an increasing sophistication in the ways of Washington and a vast army of well-financed lobbyists. Many of these lobbyists were former members of Congress or former government agency officials who knew how to get things done or, as was shortly to be the case, not get things done. When President Bill Clinton and his wife, Hillary, attempted to enact their version of health care reform, the measure was essentially dead on arrival in Congress (it never even got a floor vote).

There was a lot wrong with what opponents derided as "Hillarycare," as well as with the secretive way it was developed and arrogant manner in which it was presented. Long (1,364 pages) and exceedingly complex, the proposed legislation was an easy target for a coalition of insurance companies, Big Pharma, hospital chains, the AMA and others who sent it down in flames with a hugely expensive lobbying and advertising campaign remembered for TV commercials depicting a fictional middle-aged couple (Harry and Louise) fretting about a big government bureaucracy controlling their access to health care. Another attempt at comprehensive reform, albeit a deeply flawed one, had failed and health care was firmly in the grip of for-profit corporations whose primary goal was stockholder wealth, not patient health.

Perhaps emboldened by their success at turning back the Clintons, the health care industry expended a considerable amount of effort throughout the 1990s attempting to legitimize the idea that the for-profit model was the best approach to health care. Health care was a "privilege" earned by those who could afford it, not a right. Lofty executive pay packages were justified and health care industry CEOs were lionized as astute managers grappling with extraordinarily complex issues. Stocks continued to march upward, ultimately reaching astonishing valuations as the dot-com bubble expanded. The economy, the stock market, and even society as a whole were said to be governed by a "new paradigm". Getting rich was what really mattered.

With the medical-industrial complex actively promoting this mindset, it should have been no surprise that health care costs began to rise again. In response, many employers began to cut back and sometimes eliminate the health care coverage they had provided their employees. The number of uninsured and underinsured Americans, employed or not, rose steadily. (The percentage of underinsured and uninsured Americans today – about 15% of the population – is pretty close to what it was just before Medicare/Medicaid was enacted, meaning that we have made essentially no progress in this area.) As the 20th Century came to a close, the U.S. health care system was in dire and worsening condition.

The year 2000 saw the election of George W. Bush, who also believed deeply in the primacy of free markets. Although soon pre-occupied with other matters, the Bush Administration partnered with Big Pharma and insurance industry lobbyists, while also winning the support of the highly influential senior organization AARP, to achieve (barely) passage of the Medicare Modernization Act of 2003. The act, which took effect in 2006, created for the first time a prescription drug benefit (Medicare Part D) while also encouraging Medicare patients to switch to private managed care plans funded by Medicare (Medicare Advantage).

In acting to help Medicare patients with the costs of prescription drugs, the Bush Administration was addressing an area of major concern to seniors. There was no drug benefit in the original Medicare law enacted in 1965, in part because there weren't that many drugs available to seniors – or anyone else, for that matter. (For example, there are today more prescription medications available for cardiac care alone than the entire drug formulary that existed when I graduated from medical school.)

In the case of seniors, there have been major advances in drug therapies that have ameliorated some of the physical and mental difficulties that accompany growing old. Many seniors today routinely take a number of expensive prescription drugs, and the Medicare Modernization Act law helped them. Drugs have become a significant, and fast-growing, component of overall health care costs and now account for about 12% of those costs.

That percentage seems likely to continue rising, as does the tab for Medicare Part D. The cost, projected originally at $400 billon over 10 years, was revised shortly after passage of the Act to $530 billion. A distinctive feature of the legislation, one bearing the fingerprints of health care industry lobbyists, was that it expressly prohibited Medicare from using its clout to bargain with Big Pharma over the prices it would pay for drugs, even though other government entities such as the Veterans Administration and the Armed Forces are allowed to negotiate on drugs they buy. Moreover, instead of Medicare handling the prescription drug benefit directly, administration of the program was outsourced to private insurance companies. Investors saw the handwriting on the wall, and stocks of drug and insurance companies rose sharply as soon as the new benefit became law. Another important component of health care, prescription drugs, had joined hospitals, medical equipment manufacturers, insurers, HMOs, and others in the category of patient necessities that delivered government-guaranteed profits to profit-driven companies.

• • •

I have presented this brief history of American health care because I believe it's important as a foundation for understanding the forces that have invaded and badly damaged both the doctor-patient relationship, which I believe to be the cornerstone of health care, and the house of medicine itself. This was not the intent of the people who set these forces loose, many of whom were sincerely attempting to remedy the problems they perceived in how health care was delivered and financed. But like others before them, these people and their efforts fell victim to the Law of Unintended Consequences. What they hoped would happen did not; things they never envisioned happening did. Often, their tinkering made things worse, and the health care "system" we have today is not a system at all but instead a sputtering, patched-together contraption that is clearly in need of a major overhaul. What form that overhaul takes, a complex and divisive issue that is a central concern of the Obama Administration, is of critical importance to all of us.

Some of the things I have mentioned happened long ago, and it's fair for you to ask why they still matter. My answer is that they matter because they created the health care labyrinth in which we find ourselves today. Those of us who have tried to make things better are constantly encountering roadblocks that make no sense, entering blind alleys, and bumping up against powerful forces that stymie our progress. I do believe there is a way out, but it requires understanding what we are up against, as well as how and why things came to be the way they are. That's why I asked you to take this little dose of history.

Chapter Three

THE DOCTOR-PATIENT RELATIONSHIP IS IN CRITICAL CONDITION

How the Most Important Component of Health Care Was Lost

A pleasant little lady I'll call Ida Brown got on a train for St. Louis after visiting her children in Alabama. When she arrived home, Ida was blind, and she became my patient.

Ida went to the emergency room at the City Hospital of St. Louis, which admitted her and sent her to the floor where I worked during my junior year in medical school. In those days, medical students, acting under the supervision of a resident physician and a faculty member, commonly looked after indigent patients.

For the next three months, I was Ida's primary caretaker as we struggled to determine what had caused her sudden onset of blindness. I drew blood from her frail arms almost every day, administering every test we had, some more than once, to no avail. Through it all, she never complained but I grew increasingly frustrated at not being able to help her. Ida was always pleasant, always believed in me despite my inability to tell her why she had been struck blind.

Like many teaching hospitals, City Hospital of St. Louis periodically had what were called "Grand Rounds," where the various department heads would review patient cases. I was asked to present a patient to the Chief of Internal Medicine, Dr. Thomas Frawley, and I chose Ida. With her listening, I described her condition and the steps we had taken to find its cause. Dr. Frawley zeroed in quickly, asking Ida if she had ever had an episode of being intensely thirsty which appeared suddenly and just as suddenly disappeared. She said yes, for about three days before she got on the train.

Dr. Frawley immediately diagnosed Ida as either having lost blood supply to her hypothalamus or having a tumor in that area, this rendering her pituitary gland nonfunctional and damaging the optical nerves that wrap around the pituitary. Her episode of thirstiness, itself prompted by the malfunctioning pituitary, was the tipoff. I was stunned that anyone could possess that much knowledge, but another series of tests proved that Dr. Frawley was correct.

We couldn't cure Ida's blindness, but now that we knew what was wrong, we were able to treat the hormone deficiency caused by her malfunctioning pituitary, help her with some related problems and send her home.

Ida's story illustrates the uncertainty that often accompanies the encounter between patient and physician. She had no idea what had caused her blindness and, until Dr. Frawley's diagnosis, neither did I. But like thousands of other patients I have treated, Ida put herself in my hands, trusting that I would do my best to help her. She believed, correctly, that I had empathy for her, and that led her to trust me.

These interpersonal qualities – empathy on the part of the physician and trust on the part of the patient – make the doctor-patient relationship something very unique and very precious. Combined with what is often at stake for the patient, they also utterly differentiate the "transaction" between doctor and patient from any other type of purchase and take the doctor-patient relationship out of the realm of free markets.

Ida could not, by herself, make an informed choice on how best to respond medically to her sudden blindness. To varying degrees, most patients face the same dilemma. The notion that the core principles of free markets can function in health care ignores this reality. Although it's politically fashionable these days to suggest that societal challenges are best solved by market forces, that approach simply doesn't work in health care.

Consider for a moment the enormously dependent and vulnerable position of patients who come to a physician for the treatment of something significant, or even something minor that they fear could be something significant. In most cases, the patient has never purchased the "product" before, nor does he or she wish to sample it ahead of time. There are no guarantees, nor can the treatment be returned and the money refunded if the patient doesn't like the results. Not infrequently, patients must make choices while in pain and distress, and their decisions directly impact the most valuable thing they have – their health. In such circumstances, the rules of the marketplace must be set aside in favor of a relationship based on empathy and trust.

This is not to suggest that patients should be passive, or not try to learn everything they can about their specific situation as well as the physician who will treat them. But although this is difficult for most patients to accept, medicine is ultimately about probabilities, not certainties, and the ground is ever-changing. Even Dr. Frawley would have acknowledged that there was much he didn't know in medicine, and much has been learned in the intervening 40 years.

At some point, even the most well-informed and assertive patients are going to have to place their well-being in the hands of another, which they cannot and will not do without trust. Hopefully, they can trust the doctor who is treating them. Ida trusted me. She didn't have to, but she did and I loved her for it, wanting above all to find the cause of her illness and treat it.

As we know, trust is something that generally develops over time, which is one reason why having a long-term relationship with a primary care physician – what is now being called a "medical home" – is so important for patients. Unfortunately, this cornerstone of health care has been steadily undermined and devalued over the past 40 years – to the great detriment of individual patients and health care as a whole.

In discussing the doctor-patient relationship, I am talking about the relationship between a patient and his or her primary care physician, not a specialist. For reasons I will set forth later, the vast majority of specialists treat *diseases*, not patients. This narrow frame of reference is a critical difference that I believe has actually damaged the overall quality of American health care, while simultaneously helping to push our health care costs to unsustainable levels. Specialists have contributed significantly to improvements in medicine, but that said, we have made a grave error in allowing them to essentially define what constitutes quality in our health care system.

While Dr. Frawley's specialized knowledge of endocrinology proved to be very important to Ida, he didn't love Ida. He was in and out of her life in minutes. Dr. Frawley's contribution – and this is the appropriate function of medical specialists – was as "the doctor's doctor". I needed him as a consultant to help me help Ida. Without denigrating his contribution or expertise, Dr. Frawley was akin to a test that could divine the cause of Ida's blindness. She needed me to take the next step of treating her illness.

To the inevitable charge that I overvalue and favor primary care physicians because I am one, it just isn't true. I have always been quick to recognize when a patient needed treatment beyond my capacity to provide. I also am fully aware and greatly appreciative of the enormous advances medical science has made during the past 40-plus years as a result of specialists and their research efforts. But because I have worked inside the health care system for all that time, in many different capacities, I also am not over-awed by specialists or technology. They have their places in health care, and they are very valuable places, but we have elevated both scientists and technology to positions they don't deserve.

Because medicine is far too broad and complex for any one doctor to comprehend in its entirety, we need specialists as tools to find ways to help primary care physicians treat patients. But as many patients who encounter the impersonality of specialists learn to their dismay, the capacities of dispassionate scientist and empathetic caregiver are rarely found in the same person.

To better understand why the primary care physician is so important, let's go back to the doctor-patient relationship, to why and how a medical encounter begins. Although _how_ patients access health care is a key issue, let's leave it aside for now and look just at what actually happens in the examining room. Here are some of the ways these encounters occur.

If there is an existing relationship between doctor and patient, the examining room encounter takes place in an environment of substantial awareness on the part of the doctor as to what this patient is like. The doctor has a medical history, knows how the patient has behaved and responded in prior instances of illness or injury, knows whether the patient tends to exaggerate or downplay symptoms, knows how likely the patient is to comply with a course of treatment – in short, the doctor has a "feel" for the patient.

All that is missing when there is no existing relationship, and this emptiness must be filled with something else. Quite often that means superfluous tests, excessive caution (defensive medicine) on the part of the doctor, an over-reliance on technology, and usually a delay in getting to the root of whatever problems the patient may have.

I say "may have" because although people go to the doctor because they think something is wrong with them physically, quite often there is nothing wrong with them physically at all. There's no way to pin this down exactly, but most experts who have looked at this behavior believe that as many as half of the encounters between patient and doctor stem primarily or secondarily from mental health issues on the part of the patient. Any family doctor will tell you that many of the patients who come in, and it's often the same ones repeatedly, are really suffering from anxiety, either because of something specific that's going on in their lives or because of the existential angst that sometimes affects us all. The patient isn't sick, he or she is worried sick, or has worried a minor issue into a major "illness". This is not to make light of their situation – they are ill and the need help. Unfortunately, the health care professional who may be best able to provide that help – their family physician – is rarely able to stop and deal with a complex combination of physical and mental distress. Our nation's reimbursement system simply doesn't allow it.

This also is an area where the vast amount of information available on the Internet can make things worse. While it's wise to learn about your disease, today's patients often arrive at the doctor's office for their first visit carrying printouts from various irrelevant websites and demand to see a specialist. When they have good health care coverage, moral hazard sometimes kicks in (they're not paying; the insurance company is) and the pressure to give them what they are convinced they need can be overwhelming for a physician who has no prior relationship with the patient.

So that's one group of patients – the worried sick, who too often wind up traipsing around from one specialist to another, which of course feeds their anxiety. The majority of them would be better off with a family physician and/or a mental health professional who could help them focus on why they are so worried and what might be done about it. Once they enter what all too often becomes a forest of confusing, inconclusive and expensive tests, they really are lost.

There's another subset among those who fill doctors' waiting rooms, and that's patients whose ailments are lifestyle-related. If you smoke, drink too much, eat too much and/or unwisely, sit around too much, or engage in various other high-risk behaviors, you're going to have health problems. Doctors see such patients every day, and once again physicians have the choice of grappling with the real issues or pulling out a prescription pad, ordering tests, or handing the patient off to a specialist whose response is likely to be a highly reimbursed procedure. Adding to the dilemma is the reality that these types of patients are usually resistant, sometimes extremely so, to suggestions that they take responsibility for their own health and change their lifestyle. It's a lot easier and quicker for the doctor to prescribe a pill (today's patients, conditioned by massive pharmaceutical industry advertising, will often ask for a specific medication by name), or do something else to move the patient on. Again, even though the family physician's office is the setting in which lifestyle change is best discussed and preventive care is best delivered, our health care system's financial incentives are structured to penalize the doctor who takes time to really engage these patients and try to get them to modify their behaviors.

Of course, there are also patients who really do need the expertise of a specialist, sometimes more than one. However, as I know from first-hand experience and as many studies have shown, patients receiving specialized treatment do far better when their care is managed and coordinated by their primary care physician before and after the specialist's contribution have been made. Dr. Frawley helped me with Ida, but I was the best person to coordinate her overall treatment because we had developed a relationship and I cared about her.

The relationships I developed with my patients over the many years I practiced as a family physician were based on mutual respect and an intimate knowledge of each patient. When a worried mother called me at midnight, I would usually know just by her tone of voice how sick her child was. And because I had treated, and often delivered, her children, I knew their medical histories as well. Whatever the specific medical issue was, it came to me in a broader context that enabled me to diagnose and respond with confidence. I also knew that the mother would not abuse our relationship by calling after hours unless the problem was significant. I had taught her, if she needed to be taught, how to protect and care for her children. Our relationship was built on love, trust and her ability to depend on me absolutely when it mattered. We honored each other's right to privacy, but we also could act as if joined at the hip when it was necessary.

Because we had ongoing relationships, when my patients needed specialized care I was able to help manage and coordinate that care because I knew them. I knew when a recommended course of treatment might conflict with something else that was already going on with them. I had a good idea of how compliant a patient would be with something unpleasant. In short, I knew them and saw them as people, not as charts or diseases. This is what having a medical home is all about.

Contrast this now with the situation you will find every night in Emergency Rooms across the country. Worried patient and harried physician meet, for the first time, and in a tense and often chaotic atmosphere the doctor must try to solve the puzzle the patient presents. Sometimes the answer is apparent, but often it is not, and because of the absence of context, the always lurking issue of malpractice, and the way medical students are taught today, all too often the doctor's response is to start ordering tests instead of doing a thorough history and physical and really treating the patient. The name of the game is to move that patient along, either admitting them to the hospital (ERs are a major supply point of patients for hospitals) or, if their condition is not serious, discharging them quickly to make room for the next patient. Either way, the physician is not really "connecting" with the patient.

Our ERs are overcrowded because of a number of factors that are distorting the ways by which patients access medical care. Among these factors are the underpayment of busy primary care physicians, a reimbursement system that pays hospitals more for providing a given service than a physician who provides the exact same service, an overall squeeze on health care expenditures that has turned hospitals and physicians into competitors, and the increased use of ancillary services at hospitals.

All these developments have contributed to the disappearance of the medical home, and this absence is not going to be filled by the proliferation of Urgent Care and "Doc-in-the-Box" facilities springing up across the country. These types of facilities, which hire less qualified personnel, are structured primarily to serve the goals of their corporate owners, not the patients who come to them. In order to be able to charge less, they pay their staffers less, making up the difference on lab fees and other services (ever wonder why many of these facilities are located in or next to pharmacies?). They are a manifestation of the unmet need for ambulatory care, not a solution to it.

There's no individual villain here – patients just want to feel better, and physicians are working in an environment and under rules and incentives set by those whose objectives are not optimal health care but minimal cost and maximum incomes. Because of this, our current system's incentives are to whisk the patient into a physical diagnosis and treatment process rather than tend to his or her real needs. Because of how our health care reimbursement system has been politicized and manipulated, a talented, honest diagnostician makes much less than doctors who shoehorn patients into a Diagnostic Related Group and admit them to a hospital, order up a series of tests, or generate procedures with high reimbursements. And because primary care physicians make far less money than specialists, we have far too few of them (and the trends are discouraging, with debt-burdened medical students increasingly choosing lucrative sub-specialties rather than family medicine). This shortage of primary care physicians in turn makes it even harder for patients to access the health care system, leading them instead to the ERs and other facilities I have just mentioned. It's a vicious cycle, and it's getting worse – rapidly.

Another failing of the current system is that health care coverage is generally job-based. This means patients can easily lose their family doctor if they change jobs or their employer changes health plans. And because Medicare and most insurers don't recognize the value of a medical home and won't reimburse primary care physicians for managing and coordinating care, patients are too often left to fend for themselves. Because they don't have a medical home, patients react by ignoring their symptoms, by going to the internet, to ERs and Urgent Care centers, and to specialists they choose themselves, often using dubious parameters.

You might ask: "Don't doctors' offices transfer the records when patients move to another physician? Don't specialists check a patient's chart before beginning a course of treatment? Don't the medical professionals treating the same patient exhibit some baseline level of cooperation?" They certainly should, but what I can tell you is that so-called "handoff" issues – coordinating care when patients move among doctors and in out of hospitals and nursing homes – are a major source of quality problems in health care.

Having a medical home is all the more important when the patient has one or more chronic illnesses, which is often the case among the elderly, whose numbers are about to rise significantly as the Baby Boomers enter retirement. The American Academy of Family

Physicians estimates that more than 80% of Medicare beneficiaries have at least one chronic condition, with two-thirds having more than one and about 20% suffering from five or more chronic conditions. This 20% accounts for two-thirds of all Medicare spending.

On an individual basis, having a medical home makes it easier for patients to participate in the treatment and management of their disease(s). It helps ensure that each patient's specific medical history is taken into account when clinical decisions are made about their treatment. It promotes organized and coordinated delivery of that treatment, and, when appropriate, it helps patients deal with their diseases on an ongoing basis by providing them with links to specialists and community support groups. On a macro basis, enabling more patients to have a medical home would improve overall health care quality and cost-effectiveness. This isn't theory – it's been demonstrated by numerous studies, not to mention common sense.

The enormous advances made in science and technologies over the past four decades are miraculous. However, as measured by most parameters for the majority of patients, the overall quality of health care is not as good as it was when I graduated from medical school, a time when primary care and the medical home were the rule and not the exception.

What we see time and again in surveys of patients is that they love their primary care physician (if they have one), but think the health care system as a whole stinks. And you know what? They're right.

Unfortunately, providing a majority of patients with medical homes that would coordinate their medical care simply isn't going to happen under our current system. Although the concept has been endorsed by the Institute of Medicine and the Medicare Payment

Advisory Commission, among others, those who hold the levers of power have different priorities. As I will demonstrate in the next chapter, American health care is now about profits, not patients. The doctor-patient relationship is in critical condition, and unless we take steps to resuscitate it, we have very little chance of improving the quality of our health care system nor of reining in its runaway costs.

Chapter Four

HOW OUR PROFIT-DRIVEN HEALTH CARE SYSTEM CORRUPTS MEDICAL DECISION-MAKING

What Goes on Behind the Scenes, and How It Can Hurt Your Health

"Profit is not the explanation, cause, or rationale of business behavior and business decisions, but rather the test of their validity… Profits are really a by-product of doing business well and not the moral aim of business." – Peter Drucker

In 2003, my sons Mike and Sam and I relocated to the small California town of Turlock, where my son Joe and his partner, Dr. Bill Anderson, my daughter Lisa and then son-in-law Eric McMillan already had medical practices. We decided we now had enough Romeos and McMillans in one place to form a "federation" of small group practices and construct an office building to house them. After drawing up plans and starting construction of a full-service medical office mall, which we named the Tower Health and Wellness Center (www.tower-health.com), we began to think about the equipment we would need. At this point, our group, like the many thousands of small medical groups that deliver some 70% of American health care, faced a decision that I believe illustrates the perverse and potentially corrupting influences our health care system exerts on those who work within it.

Among the many equipment purchases we considered was a Magnetic Resonance Imaging (MRI) scanner, a useful but extremely expensive diagnostic tool. A scanner would have been very helpful to Dr. Sam, Dr. Mike, and Drs. Eric and Lisa, and to a lesser degree to others in our federation. But since this would be a major capital investment, we needed to weigh the costs and benefits carefully.

We contacted General Electric, a major manufacturer of MRI scanners, and they sent out a salesman. He was most helpful, presenting us with a detailed business plan that showed us exactly how many scans we would need to do to break even, and how much we would make at varying numbers of scans above that point. Everything was figured in – installation costs, monthly payments, depreciation, salaries for technicians, etc. – as well as how much revenue would be generated by different volumes of MRIs.

The salesman was able to compute those revenue figures because reimbursements from payers to providers for MRIs are fixed – we would get essentially the same amount from an insurer every time we turned on the machine. In most other industries, prices drop as volume increases – 1,000 computers cost less per unit than four – but it doesn't work that way in health care. MRI scans, like thousands of other procedures, are reimbursed at fixed rates set by the government and private insurers.

Because of this, our decision on whether or not to buy the scanner (generous financing was available from GE) was fairly straightforward, based really on one question. How many scans did we think we would do a year? Too few and we would have trouble making the payments on the scanner; quite a few and we would turn a nice profit.

Turlock has about 70,000 people, which by our estimates meant that the number patients we would be seeing who needed MRIs in the ordinary course of events would not be sufficient to justify purchasing the scanner. On the other hand, since we would be the ones recommending (which essentially means deciding) whether this or that patient "needed" an MRI, we could nudge that number higher if we so chose.

A scanner can be very helpful to a medical group, facilitating diagnoses and generally helping the practice to operate more efficiently. Patients who get MRIs also may view their treatment – and therefore their doctor – as more thorough and caring. A scanner also can be a significant source of revenue, an especially meaningful consideration for hard-pressed primary care physicians whose income is far lower than that of specialists. These factors can make it tempting for physicians to order more MRIs than their patients really need. It's a slippery slope, greased in part by the perception that someone else – not the patient, but the patient's insurer – is paying (moral hazard again).

We didn't buy the scanner. It simply wasn't the right thing to do.

I cite this example not to appear holier-than-thou nor to trumpet the ethical values of my family, but to illustrate how the reimbursement structure of American health care – and particularly the profit motive and margins embedded in that structure – have come to drive, and often to undermine, medical decision-making.

Many other medical groups have made different choices than we did, and you can see the results in the statistics on MRI usage. Medicare's outlays for imaging services more than doubled between 2000 and 2005 – from $6.6 billion to $13.7 billion – and have continued to grow. Some portion of this increase no doubt is legitimate – MRIs can be very valuable diagnostically. But some of the increase has occurred because physicians are sending their patients to imaging centers the physicians own – a practice known as self-referral. The federal Centers for Medicare and Medicaid Services say self-referral arrangements are "creating incentives for over-utilization and corrupting medical decision-making."

Why is this (and other variations on the same theme) happening? The convenient, simplistic answer is "greedy doctors," but I believe that the real problem runs much deeper. Our society has come to glorify and worship wealth above all else, an enormously destructive development whose manifestations can be seen in everything from obscenely over-compensated CEOs to sneakers that cost $250. The distinction between "needs" and "wants" has been obliterated, and whatever moral compass we may once have had is no longer functioning. When people whose God is money get hold of the levers of a $2 trillion machine (what we're spending on health care) with inexhaustible demand, the results range from the $6 aspirin on your hospital bill to the $1.5 billion that Dr. William McGuire received as the head of United Healthcare. What does it say about our values as a society when McGuire, who resigned in 2006 amidst a controversy about manipulated stock options, can take home this kind of money while many family physicians can't make a living?

Basic health care is a need, not a want, and as such it must be addressed within the context of moral and ethical considerations. But because health care is a need, and sometimes a very pressing need, it can be easily exploited by those who care only about profits. What's happened to us – partially because American medical care is delivered within the framework of the haphazard, patched-together "system" I described in Chapter Two and partially because materialism has triumphed over morality – is that health care has become a "growth industry" rather than a societal need. If the Robber Barons of the early 1900s were operating today, they'd be in health care.

Before going any further, let me say that I believe deeply in both free markets and the profits that can be earned within them. Truly free markets are a wonderful mechanism for encouraging innovation, eliminating inefficiency and waste, creating value and wealth, and fostering individual upward mobility. Profits, as management authority Peter Drucker says, are a legitimate byproduct of operating a business well. And there's nothing inherently wrong with individuals and companies making as much as they can – *as long as they are operating in the area of wants*. But there's something very wrong when that happens in the area of needs. It was wrong for Enron to gouge consumers of energy, and it's wrong for those who operate within health care system to exploit that system and the patients who depend on it.

I feel I need to set out this disclaimer because those who criticize the vast and powerful for-profit health care industry – which includes publicly held HMOs, hospital chains, insurance companies, big pharmaceutical companies, and various other players – are often characterized as being "against free markets". The not-too-subtle suggestion accompanying this charge is that if you are "against free markets," you are also somehow anti-American. The medical-industrial complex in general, and Big Pharma in particular, are especially good at this. They brush aside criticism by claiming that without free markets there will be no incentives to innovate and develop new drugs, technologies and procedures that can save lives and improve people's health.

This is a smokescreen. Remember the CEOs of the major tobacco companies who lined up in a Congressional hearing and said, under oath and with straight faces, that they did not believe cigarette smoking was addictive? Executives of for-profit, publicly traded health care companies who talk about the virtues of free markets in health care are engaging in the same kind of lying, manipulative behavior. They know perfectly well that health care is not a free market; in fact, they depend on it not being a free market. Their business models and strategies are built essentially on two factors – people will always need health care and the prices they pay for it can be manipulated.

As I've discussed earlier, health care is not a free market because people don't choose to be ill or injured. Those who need health care, especially those who need it urgently, are in an unwilling and vulnerable position where they generally can neither evaluate the supplier (physicians and other health care providers) nor bargain on prices. But it's also not a free market because prices – like those for MRI scans – are primarily fixed by forces external to the market, namely by Medicare and insurers following Medicare's lead.

How do Medicare and other payers arrive at these prices? In the case of treatment delivered within a physician's office, a given procedure is identified by what is known as its CPT© code – for Current Procedural Terminology. The little boxes your doctor checks off on a sheet at the end of your office visit are

CPT© codes (more on this in the next chapter). Because every procedure has a code and a corresponding reimbursement level, revenue to a provider essentially becomes a function of volume. This is why the friendly MRI salesman was able to tell us with a fairly high degree of accuracy how much we would make if we did 200 scans a month, or 300, or 400.

Now, this being health care, things are a little more complicated. In another distortion, everyone doesn't pay the same price. If you work for a big company that has a good health plan, a procedure with a nominal price of $3,000 might be negotiated down to maybe $600, and your copay might be somewhere between $10 and $30. If you work for a small company, as most employees do, the health plan, if there is one, probably won't be as good. If you work a minimum-wage, service-industry job, which means you really need help with health care expenses, it's highly unlikely that you have health insurance, which means that your price is the "sticker price" of $3,000, the steepest of all. In other words, those with the least resources often pay the highest prices. This is the plight of the millions of uninsured in the U.S. and the reason that a major illness often forces uninsured or under-insured people into bankruptcy.

From an economics standpoint, the important point here is that there is no *price transparency*, which is another component of free markets. When you drive past a gas station and see the prices for various grades of gasoline, that's price transparency. You can argue that those prices are too high, and they may well be, but at least you know what you're going to pay for a gallon of high-test. You also can respond to your perception, by buying a car with better mileage, riding your bike or taking the bus. What do you do when you need an appendectomy?

Price transparency and price competition do appear in health care categories where Medicare and insurers won't pay. Take LASIK surgery, which generally isn't covered by insurance, or covered only minimally. Open up your newspaper, especially the health or wellness section, or watch your local TV channel for a while and you're likely to find LASIK centers advertising their procedures for $599 an eye, maybe less. They're competing on price, just as a car dealer or termite company or massage therapist or other business might. The same phenomenon is true for various types of elective/cosmetic plastic surgery such as hair transplants, breast augmentation and so on. The free market is at work, and prices are competitive as a result. Please note that I am not suggesting that price alone is the best criterion for making decisions on your health care – you don't necessarily want the cheapest cardiologist or neurosurgeon in town. But price matters, and it matters a lot more to those without health insurance than those with it.

About that insurance. Let's take a step back for a moment and consider what's going on with most of the types of insurance we buy, and what's going on with health insurance. When you buy auto, home or life insurance, you're seeking to protect yourself against something you hope won't happen – a car accident, a kitchen fire, a fatal heart attack. Health insurance is a somewhat different animal. We expect it to protect us from financial ruin in the case of things we hope won't happen – a major illness – but we also expect it to cover us in the case of things we know <u>will</u> happen – pregnancies, flu, sprained ankles, etc.

Insurance companies are very good at figuring out how many car accidents are likely to occur in any given year for a particular category of drivers, say those aged 40-50 with no accidents or tickets in the past five years. Auto insurance companies spread the risk they are taking on among a pool of drivers, determine their premiums according to the company's calculations of what it's likely to have to pay out and what it can earn on the money taken in before it's paid out, and present you with a price quote. As I'm sure you know, they compete on price, often ferociously.

Health insurance is a lot trickier, which is why commercial insurers stayed away from it until prices became fixed through Medicare and the related mechanisms I will discuss in this book. But it's still pretty tricky, because health care expenses can be open-ended, especially for certain illnesses. So insurance companies exclude, either overtly or covertly, those people whose health profiles make them likely to be losing propositions for the company. Good luck getting individual health insurance if you have diabetes. Remember moral hazard? – "I don't care what it costs because my insurance is paying". Here it is in reverse – "We'll pay for your health care needs as long as we can make money on you, but if you have a medical condition where we might lose money, we won't take you". This practice, known as medical underwriting, essentially means that insurers are writing their policies to protect themselves from having to protect you.

The net result of what might be described as dueling moral hazard is that customer and company wind up as adversaries instead of cooperating to meet each other's needs. There's nothing wrong with health insurance companies making a profit on their operations, but there's something terribly wrong when that's accomplished by denying legitimate claims.

Let's step back even further for a moment and think about the way most Americans get their health insurance (if they have it), which is through their employer. As I explained in Chapter Two, this is essentially an historical accident – an unintended consequence of the wage controls imposed on employers during World War II and solidified by IRS rulings that allowed companies to deduct health insurance as a business expense. But because job-based health insurance has become the de facto "system," most people really don't question it or think about whether a different approach might serve everyone better. As I asked earlier, would you let your employer decide where you could live or what kind of car you could drive? Not likely. So why are we letting employers choose something as critically important as our health insurance? Why are we allowing employers to decide (which they do when they select the health plans they offer) which doctors we can see?

As noted above, those who work for big companies generally have a wider range of choices when it comes to health insurance, with those choices dwindling for employees of smaller companies (the bulk of all workers) and often vanishing for those who work in the lowest-paid jobs. In other words, the *size* of your employer dictates how good your health insurance is. Does that seem like a good idea? Does it sound like a free market?

So if American health care is not a free market, and I think I have convincingly demonstrated that it is not, then what is it? My answer is that it's a jungle, a no-holds barred free-for-all with Alice in Wonderland logic where the prevailing value system is "I'm going to get mine." While this attitude reflects our larger societal problem of glorifying wealth, the issue is particularly pernicious in health care because we're dealing with the most precious thing a person has. It's one thing to get your Learjet by persuading consumers to buy blue jeans with metal spangles and a designer label; it's something very different when patients' best interests are subordinated to profits.

Behind the smokescreen of "free markets" are numerous examples of profits trumping patients in every sector of health care. Let's start with a hospital chain now called Tenet Healthcare, which in 2004 paid $54 million to settle charges brought by federal prosecutors that hundreds of patients at a Tenet hospital in Northern California had endured cardiac surgeries that they didn't need – with Medicare, Medicaid and other government programs receiving fraudulent bills for the procedures. Shortly after settling with the government, Tenet also settled with the victims and their families, paying them $395 million. The four surgeons who had operated on the patients also agreed to multi-million penalties in accompanying civil suits.

It's important to understand how the suit-and-settlement game works, because in the case of for-profit health care companies with their legions of slick lawyers, you almost never get a crystal-clear "smoking gun" example of illegal activity. Companies like Tenet, and others I will cite, readily spend many, many millions of dollars to defend themselves in cases like this and, when their backs are against the wall, they settle "without admitting wrongdoing." In many instances, prosecutors are simply out-gunned by high-priced legal teams and make the tactical decision to "send a message" to the industry by punishing the company financially. The corporation, on the other hand, generally sees all this as simply another cost of doing business. The legal fees spent on battling the case in court are deductible expenses and when it's all said and done, guess who pays the bill (wonder why your hospital aspirin costs $6?). Their expenses become our costs. In some cases, notably Enron, prosecutors do send people to jail, but it's still true that if you're going to live a life of crime, be sure you're wearing a white collar and know how to operate a shredder.

So, without being able to prove it beyond a shadow of a doubt, here is what evidence gathered by the FBI from cardiologists in the area said about Tenet's Redding Medical Center and its heart surgeons: As many as half of the 1,000 cardiac procedures (in a 238-bed hospital) done over the course of a year were "unnecessary by commonly held medical standards" and about one-quarter were done on patients who had no serious heart problems at all. Some of these folks died.

An isolated instance? I don't think so. In a previous incarnation 10 years earlier as National Medical Enterprises, the same company paid a (then) record $379 million in fines and pleaded guilty to eight criminal counts in a 30-state case that involved bribing high school counselors and doctors to refer adolescent patients to company-owned psychatric hospitals where they were held against their will until their insurance ran out.

Was Tenet/National Medical Enterprises just a bad apple in an otherwise honest hospital industry? It doesn't seem so. HCA (a mammoth hospital chain created by the merger of Columbia Healthcare Corporation and Hospital Corporation of America) pleaded guilty in 2000 to more than a dozen felonies and wound up paying some $1.7 billion in civil and criminal fines. Among the charges: HCA had paid kickbacks to physicians to steer patients to the company's hospitals and defrauded Medicare with bogus billings that included such items as $18,000 for liquor. HCA, it turned out, had kept two sets of books. In another case, HealthSouth, the nation's largest chain of rehabilitation hospitals, paid $325 million to settle claims of Medicare fraud.

Just hospitals? Well, no. Ever wonder how your orthopedic surgeon decided which artificial hip or knee to put in as a replacement when that joint gave out? Maybe he or she carefully considered all the competing devices available and made an impartial decision based on which one was best for you. Then again, maybe not. The four largest manufacturers of artificial hips and knees agreed in late 2007 to pay a total of $311 million to settle criminal and civil investigations into allegations that they paid kickbacks to surgeons who used their products. Along with a fifth company that cooperated with prosecutors and agreed to corporate monitoring for 18 months, these firms account for almost 95% of knee and hip replacements sold in the U.S.

The beat goes on. WellPoint Inc., a publicly traded insurance company headquartered in Indiana, persuaded California regulators late in 2004 to approve its purchase of Blue Cross of California by promising to maintain and improve services to members. In 2007, the state's Department of Managed Health Care (DMHC), while citing numerous complaints from Blue Cross members, appeared to realize (belatedly) that it had been had. WellPoint, it seems, was raising premiums and cutting services while simultaneously paying itself a $950 million dividend from Blue Cross – almost twice what it pulled out in the prior two years.

"The dividend is significant because it (WellPoint) is extracting a large amount of money at the same time it is saying the increasing costs of health care require premium increases and benefit reductions," said DMHC Director Cindy Ehnes.

About the same time, Blue Cross of California paid a $1 million fine and settled a class-action suit in which it was accused of canceling individual health insurance policies when the policyholders has the temerity to file claims. Such individual policies, which in the case of Blue Cross became known as "use-it-and-lose-it" health coverage, are increasingly important in an era when many companies are cutting back on what they offer employees (about three million people in California, just to cite one state, have individual policies).

Blue Cross is not alone. In November 2007, California's DHMC fined Health Net $1 million for misleading the agency about the company's policy of linking employee bonuses to cancellations. Internal Health Net documents revealed that the company set goals for the cancellation of individual policies and rewarded employees when they met or exceeded those goals. One employee whose performance in rescinding individual policies exceeded her goals was praised by her supervisor as having a "banner year" and saving Health Net some "$6 million in unnecessary healthcare expenses." The example of this outstanding employee, who had rescinded 301 individual policies in just one year, came to light through a lawsuit filed by a hair salon owner, Patsy Bates, who said she was left with nearly $200,000 in medical bills when Health Net rescinded her policy while she was undergoing chemotherapy for breast cancer. Bates' case went before an arbitration judge, who ruled in her favor early in 2008 and hit Health Net with a $9.4 million penalty, of which $8.4 million was punitive damages.

"Health Net was primarily concerned with and considered its own financial interests and gave little, if any, consideration and concern for the interests of the insured," the arbitration judge, Sam Cianchetti, wrote in his ruling. "It's difficult to imagine a policy more reprehensible than tying bonuses to encourage the rescission of health insurance that keeps the public well and alive."

Health Net says it has abandoned the bonus-for-rescissions policy. But the underlying business model of publicly-held HMOs remains the same – the less they pay out, the higher their profits, which is how the management team is judged and compensated. What do you think their incentives are?

I could go on – there's no shortage of examples. Drugs that cost $300 a month in the U.S. are somehow legally available for much less in Canada (more on drug companies later on), sparking a thriving business in cross-border purchases. Nursing homes residents die as corporate owners cut expenses by laying off nurses (A New York Times analysis of Medicare/Medicaid records shows that at 60% of nursing homes bought by large private equity groups from 2000 to 2006, managers have cut the number of clinical RNs, sometimes far below levels required by law). In short, the proof that the medical-industrial complex routinely puts profits ahead of patients is no further away than your newspaper or nightly TV news. The more pressing issue is why we put up with this.

Part of the answer, I believe, lies in the displacement of the financial responsibility for our individual health care onto third-party payers – a group which includes employers, Medicare, Medicaid, the Veterans Administration, the federal government itself, and various other entities. When gasoline prices head north of $3 a gallon, it comes right out of our pockets and we get mad. When a hospital charges $6 for an aspirin, we shake our heads and shrug – after all, insurance is paying and who cares if an insurance company gets screwed? This displacement obscures and disperses our outrage. We don't really focus on the fact that we ultimately do pay for the $6 aspirin, or other expensive drug, or marked-up medical device, or executive jet. We may realize this abstractly, or bitch about our higher premiums and co-pays, but if we have decent health insurance and feel pretty safe personally, we don't really care.

Another aspect of this displacement onto third-party payers is that patients and their families have come to feel entitled to anything and everything that medicine has to offer. When Grandma gets sick, it's no longer considered to be part of the aging process and a natural prelude to death. Instead, Grandma and her family will demand every procedure in the book, and woe betide the doctor who stands in their way. In fairness, and I will talk more about this, doctors often abet this process, in part because they want to help Grandma, in part because they are paid based on what they do, but also because too many of them now see her less as a human being and more as a disease(s) to be treated.

Still another aspect of why we allow profits to prevail in healthcare is that they prevail everywhere else. We don't draw the distinctions we should with health care – it's become acceptable for there to be a "healthcare industry" and "markets" for diabetes or colon cancer. The free market myth promoted so successfully by big health care corporations has somehow veiled the fact that patients such as diabetics and colon cancer victims are essentially over a barrel when it comes to medical care. When the (health care) consumer's situation comes down to "pay or die," that's not quite the same thing as choosing cars or clothes, is it?

To reiterate, I have nothing against profits in health care, as long as ethical and moral considerations are also part of the equation. But I also believe our societal values have deteriorated significantly over the past two or three decades, to the point where it's the trappings of success that matter, not how that success was achieved. Examining the reasons for this erosion of ethics are outside the scope of this book, but I don't think there's any doubt that it has happened, and that it has happened in health care.

There are other factors in the mix. Americans love technology, and the media unquestioningly focuses on and fawns over the latest wonder drug, DNA-related discovery or complex micro-surgical procedure. And while there's no question that science has brought us astonishing advances in medicine, the big payoffs in terms of our collective health come not from technology but from unglamorous work such as efforts to reduce the obesity rate in this country. Medical technology is not only expensive, it's also extremely hard to pin down precisely in terms of costs and benefits, which enables profit-oriented corporations to reap enormous profits when they develop new procedures and prescriptions.

Finally, there is the simple fact that a great many people make their living in the health care "industry" as it is now constituted. A recent Price Waterhouse Coopers study estimated that roughly one in every eight U.S. residents has a job somehow connected to the health care system. Two trillion dollars spent every year on health care translates into a lot of jobs. Everyone from the mailroom clerk at Amgen who buys company stock for his/her pension plan, to the administrator at a Tenet hospital who get stock options, to the doctor who goes to the Bahamas courtesy of a medical manufacturer, to the CEO of WellPoint whose compensation is tied directly to corporate profits, has a vested interest in the status quo. Health care profits are woven directly into the fabric of our society, on many different levels, in many different ways. This makes it easier for people to go along with the program. When reforms are proposed, those whose living comes from health care react not in terms of whether the reform in question is good for society as a whole, but in terms of what it means to their financial situation.

If we had been able to visualize the current state of affairs in health care as a destination, I don't think any of us (or almost any) would have gone down this road. We wound up here unintentionally, without really understanding the ramifications of the choices we made along the way. But we're coming to a dead end, a system that's collapsing on our heads, and we're going to have to do something different.

Chapter Five

HOW HEALTH CARE CAME TO FOCUS ON DISEASES RATHER THAN PATIENTS

Why Doctors Can't Get Paid for Doing the Things that Would Help You the Most

One of the most unfortunate changes in American medicine over the last 40 years has been a gradual but enormously significant deterioration in the way that health care providers view the patients they treat. To put it simply, they don't see patients, they see pieces. Rather than looking at the living, breathing, feeling person before them, far too many physicians and other providers now "see" defective necks, kidneys, hearts, eyes, etc., and respond based on that perception. The impersonality, haste, and excessive expense that characterize modern health care have their roots in this "diseases-rather-than-patients" orientation.

A number of factors have contributed to this sad transition, whose effects can be seen in the mis-education of medical students, the segmentation of the physician community into specialists, distortions in the development of medical technology, and the wrong-headed reimbursement policies of government agencies and private payers. Declines in one area of health care have contributed to and fed off declines in another, and the entire House of Medicine has suffered as a result. I will deal with each of these areas in subsequent chapters, but let's start with the seemingly innocent change that set them all in motion – the development of CPT Codes.

The little boxes your doctor checks off on a form at the conclusion of your office visit are called CPT Codes – for Current Procedural Terminology (CPT®) – and they are intended to describe, in a standarized way, the treatment you received from your doctor. They also are the foundation for a complex process that determines what your doctor is going to be paid for treating you. As you can therefore imagine, they are very important. In fact, it's no exaggeration to say that American health care revolves around CPT Codes and similar coding systems intended to quantify what specific medical procedures are worth. Because CPT Codes have such a huge influence on the treatment you receive from your doctors and on our health care system in general, I ask you to stay with me for a little while as I explain how and why they originated.

The AMA created and published the first CPT Codes in 1966, the same year Medicare took effect. The first code set was concerned primarily with surgical procedures, although some other medical services also were described. The intent was to standardize the terms physicians used to describe the procedures and services they were performing. Agreed-upon descriptors, it was thought, would help government agencies and other payers to know with more precision what they were paying for, improve the overall accuracy of medical records, assist in evaluating the efficacy of surgical procedures and begin to establish a database for actuarial and statistical analysis. Later CPT editions were expanded to cover a broader range of diagnostic and therapeutic procedures, including internal medicine and the ever-increasing number of medical specialties. In the early 1980s, Medicare and Medicaid mandated the use of CPT Codes as part of their reimbursement procedures, which effectively established these codes as the language virtually all payers and providers would use to communicate with each other.

Now this being health care, it of course gets more complicated. Once your doctor checks off the little box denoting the CPT code, what he or she actually gets paid is modified based on something called the Resource-Based Relative Value Scale. Medicare, Medicaid, and virtually all other payers use the RBRVS, which originated in a Harvard University study. The RBRVS arrives at the fee to be paid the physician by multiplying the dollar amount specified for a particular CPT Code by a fixed conversion factor, which changes annually. The conversion factor takes into account the amount of work the physician did in performing the procedure (this includes the physician's time, mental effort, technical skill, judgment, stress and an amortization of the physician's education), as well as the physician's practice expense and malpractice expense. The calculation of the final fee also includes a geographic adjustment (i.e., a tonsillectomy done in San Francisco is "worth" more than one done in Turlock). The RBRVS does not include adjustments for outcomes, quality of service, severity, or demand.

Because medicine changes so rapidly, the AMA also established a regular schedule for updating the CPT Codes so that new procedures and treatments deemed worthwhile could be assigned a code and included in the overall set. This responsibility was assigned to a group called the CPT Editorial Panel, which is composed primarily of specialty physicians but also includes doctors representing Blue Cross, Blue Shield, America's Health Insurance Plans, the American Hospital Association, the Centers for Medicare and Medicaid Services (CMS), as well as advisory groups and (more recently) performance measurement advisory groups.

Under the CPT Editorial Panel are groups called the CPT Advisory Committees, again dominated by specialty physicians, that make recommendations on whether or not newly developed medical and surgical procedures should be given a CPT Code. Various other sources of information, including medical textbooks, published articles and studies, and assessments by other AMA boards, are also taken into consideration. The decisions of the CPT Editorial Panel are crucial to physicians for one simple reason: If you perform a procedure on or provide a service to a patient that isn't in the CPT code, you don't get paid. As a quick example, one reason physicians generally won't use email to receive and answer their patients' questions is that there's no way to code for it. An hour or two spent corresponding with patients is lost time financially for physicians, who have little enough time as it is. This is especially true for primary care physicians.

Measuring and improving the quality of health care has been of paramount importance to me throughout my career and I have been privileged to serve on several national organizations focused on assuring quality. Because of my background, some years ago I became part of a group advising the CPT Editorial Panel on quality measurement. As a novice in the process, and while attending a meeting of the CPT Editorial Panel as a performance measurement advisor, I attended a breakout session on how codes are developed. What I observed there reinforced what I had long believed – that new procedures are often approved primarily because they are good for physician revenue and only secondarily because they are good medicine. I said as much, and was immediately ruled out of order and essentially told to shut up by the Editorial Panel member, a surgeon, who was running the meeting. I had pointed to the elephant in the room. I'm sure I wasn't the only one who recognized what was going on, but the others didn't say anything. However, after the meeting, several people told me what I had said should be said more often.

In recounting this story, I don't mean to imply that the CPT Editorial Panel is engaging in some kind of fraud. It's not. It's fulfilling its role of evaluating new medical procedures and assigning a code to those deemed beneficial. But there is a financial subtext, and I believe it overshadows the ostensible purpose of the proceedings and in fact contributes greatly to the reality that American health care is focused on treating diseases instead of patients.

Because CPT codes and the RBRVS govern whether or not and how much a physician is reimbursed, doctors as a whole have been indoctrinated into a different mindset, with different underlying values and decision-making parameters. Here's another quick example: A physician who talks with an obese patient about diet, exercise and lifestyle changes very often cannot obtain reimbursement for that – there's no CPT code for counseling that patient on prevention and wellness. But if that same physician staples the same patient's stomach, the reimbursement is handsome indeed. Draw your own conclusions from that.

The original purpose in developing the CPT Codes was to have everyone working from the same page, which is a good idea in any endeavor but undeniably important when it comes to health care. However, as with other well-intentioned measures, this one has had a wide range of unintended consequences that have damaged the overall quality of American health care. One of the most significant has been a major shift in the priorities of physicians and a change in their ethical and social decision-making process.

As the use of CPT Codes expanded to become the gold standard (hospitals use CPT Codes to bill for outpatient care and have a similar system called Healthcare Common Procedure Coding System - HCPCS - for inpatient care), the way physicians and other providers regarded patients changed inexorably. Doctors began to think more about what they would and wouldn't do, with the logic matrix underlying those decisions affected significantly by whether a specific treatment or procedure had a CPT Code. The needs of the patient and the needs of the doctor began to diverge, with the doctor forced to balance what was best for the patient with what was necessary for the doctor to survive financially.

This was a major change, and not for the better. Financial considerations have always been present in health care, but this was something different. There was now another presence in the examining room, invisible to most patients but a force to be reckoned with for every doctor. The specific choices the doctor made in treating the patient were inevitably colored by the financial consequences of those choices. One way to conceptualize it is this: A good physician will do something that helps the patient even if there isn't a CPT Code for it; a physician whose primary orientation is financial reward will not.

There's no way to quantify what this has meant – we're talking about millions and millions of individual choices made by thousands of physicians over many years – but the cumulative effects are readily apparent in the expensive, wasteful, assembly-line health care we have today. Health care decision-making is no longer centered on what's best for patients. There are other factors, and quite often the tail wags the dog.

The patients-as-diseases-rather-than-people mindset that CPT Codes helped create has contributed greatly to a mis-allocation of effort that is driving up costs while also making it less likely that the overall health profile of Americans will improve. To explain why, I'm going to change the frame of reference and look for a moment at something else – our polluted rivers.

Cleaning up a polluted river at its mouth is enormously expensive because you have to remove all kinds of pollutants that have been dumped into the water all along its length. By the time everything is intermingled, it's extremely complicated to deal with. It's much more effective to treat each source of pollution where it originates, i.e., stopping a specific metal plating firm from dumping waste into the river upstream.

Patients are much the same way. By the time an elderly diabetic patient comes into a physician's examining room, he or she almost always has multiple, inter-related problems that are difficult and expensive to treat. The sad truth is that often these folks aren't going to get better – the physician is engaged in a holding action at best. If they could have been reached early in their lives and helped to make better choices about diet and exercise, the situation would have been much different.

The same is true for a wide variety of diseases – we can prevent them if we can educate people and persuade them to make better lifestyle choices. But guess what? Generally speaking, a physician can't code for prevention and wellness counseling. In cases where they can, the reimbursement is a tiny fraction of what coding for a specific disease such as diabetes will yield.

What this produces on a macro scale is the misallocation of effort and money I mentioned earlier. Our health care system spends an enormous amount of money on patients who are in their last six months of life and relatively little on helping young people make choices that will improve their health for decades to come. The epidemic of childhood diabetes we are seeing in this country has frightening implications, but in their roles as physicians my kids generally can't code for counseling a six-year-old and his mom about diet and exercise. By the time that patient is 50 or 60, however, one of my great-grand-children (assuming the Romeo history of becoming physicians holds true) may well be treating him or her for blindness, lost limbs, heart disease, stroke and other diabetes-related complications. Leaving compassion aside for a moment, this simply isn't efficient or cost-effective health care.

People will always have injuries and illnesses, and changing our coding procedures won't change that. But we're putting our health care emphasis and dollars in the wrong place – the mouth of the river, if you will – and that's never going to work.

The emergence of CPT Codes as the fulcrum for health care decisions also has had consequences in areas outside the examining room, and we're spending a lot of money unnecessarily there too as a result. For example, because these codes govern reimbursement, providers are forced into playing paperwork games that have nothing to do with whether or not their patients are being cared for appropriately.

Here's how this sometimes happens. When you see your family doctor, he or she can check off one of five separate CPT Codes for an office visit, starting with 99211 and ending in 99215. The higher numbers are supposed to correspond with more complex, demanding levels of service requiring more time, effort and knowledge, and if your doctor isn't able to document that, he or she could be accused of fraud. But only the doctor knows what really occurred in the examining room as far as the CPT Code is concerned, and higher numbers are reimbursed at higher rates. What's happened over the last several decades is that more and more office visits have come to be coded at 99213 and 99214 instead of 99211 and 99212. This is what's known as "code creep."

In another distortion, some physicians will try to "unbundle" the care they deliver to patients by separating treatment into as many different CPT Codes as possible and then billing the payer for each one. For example, a surgeon who can code for each action he or she takes in the course of an operation will make more than one who simply codes for, say, an appendectomy.

I believe that the primary motivation for code creep and other coding gambits was and is not greed but the ever-tighter squeeze on physicians' incomes by third-party payers. The costs of running a medical practice have risen at far greater rates than reimbursement has. This presents physicians with a stark choice – see more patients in a day (head 'em up and move 'em out) or somehow find a way to shift the same number of patients into higher codes. Ramming as many patients as possible through an eight or 10-hour day pretty much eliminates the chance for real human interaction between doctor and patient, and thereby lessens the overall quality of care. The other choice – code creep or unbundling – may be more humane as far as the patient is concerned, but the aggregate effect of thousands of physicians doing this is to drive overall health care costs higher and higher.

Trying to provide quality care while staying alive financially inevitably leads a physician onto tricky ground. There exists today within medicine an entire sub-industry composed of CPT Code specialists who work for medical practices and whose job is to maximize physician reimbursement. Similar specialists exist on the payer side (insurance companies and others) trying to minimize payments. The two armies fight it out every day, and we all end up paying the bill. Great use of human talent and financial resources, don't you think?

Another consequence of the strait-jacketing of medicine into CPT Codes is that procedures have come to be valued more highly than human interaction. For example, I could make more money doing a single hernia surgery at 6 a.m. than I would seeing 35 patients in my office during the rest of the day. Certain procedures came to be valued very highly indeed, and don't think for a second that physicians and med students didn't notice that. This has contributed to a stratification of medicine in which primary care physicians make far less than specialists, and one consequence is that we face a critical shortage of primary care physicians. Having put five kids through medical school and watched them struggle to make a living playing by the Alice-in-Wonderland reimbursement rule book that CPT Codes represent, I fully understand why most med students don't go into primary care. If you come out of school carrying substantial debt and want to be a compassionate family doctor delivering quality care, you have set yourself an almost impossible goal. I'll discuss this point in more detail shortly.

Another side effect of CPT coding, this one more subtle but certainly significant, is that an increasing amount of medical innovation is occurring abroad, not in the United States. Here's why.

Healing another person is an art as well as a science, and is likely to remain that way regardless of how many technological discoveries are made. Because of this, medicine often advances because a physician does something different – pushes the envelope, if you will. This happens with some frequency in wartime, where battlefield surgeons unencumbered by codes and reimbursement considerations reach out in the urgency of the moment and try something new. If it works, if the patient's outcome is better, the surgeon may try it again. Other surgeons take notice of the new technique – either because of direct observation, conversation, or publication – and they try it too. Over time, a new technique is developed and disseminated.

The same dynamic was present when I treated Ida Brown, the little lady who suddenly went blind. People don't always like to hear this, but a lot of medical innovation used to come out of the county hospitals where the indigent were treated. When a physician had done all the conventional, accepted treatments with a patient and wasn't getting anywhere, that physician would sometimes try something a little different. If it worked, the physician would try it again, and perhaps write it up if the success rate warranted that. Other physicians would learn of it and medicine would advance.

This happens less now, and one big reason is that today the physician couldn't code for the new procedure and therefore wouldn't get paid. There are other factors, including increased anxiety about malpractice suits, the overly tight rein the Food and Drug Administration keeps on innovation, the politicization of specialty review boards, and the dissolution of county hospitals. However, the reality that Medicare, Medicaid and private insurers won't pay for something that doesn't have a CPT Code is not lost on physicians.

The American medical establishment is too arrogant to admit it, but many of the latest medical techniques are being developed in European and Asian countries, often by physicians who trained here and then took their knowledge home where they could innovate with fewer restrictions.

The same is true for new drug therapies, which often come to light first in foreign medical journals. Overseas physicians, unfettered by restrictive pre-research agendas and with more open access to patients, are able to try drugs they couldn't use in the U.S. Our system has hemmed us in, with drugs that could help people who are desperate for help kept off the market for far longer than necessary. The next time you read a newspaper story about a promising new drug that has already helped a lot of people in several trials, there's quite likely to be a sentence noting that the drug won't be generally available for another three to five years. The mindset that CPT codes has helped create is one reason.

There are other factors in the diseases-rather-than-patients mentality, among them the increasing tendency of patients to show up at a physician's office with a firm, if sometimes ill-informed, opinion on what their course of treatment should be. Because fewer and fewer patients have a medical home, they often come in with a viewpoint based on some website, or their impression of how a neighbor was treated for a similar complaint, or their recollection of what a previous doctor did when the ailment in question surfaced some time back. Patients also are understandably anxious about health care these days, and one way to assuage that anxiety is to "take charge" of their care by telling the doctor what to do.

In a more ideal scenario, the doctor and patient would have a history together and would collaborate on how to respond to the problem. As any doctor who has been practicing for a few years will tell you, one of the best diagnostics is a little time for observation. If the doctor says, "Let's watch this for a week or so" and their prior history has engendered trust, the patient is likely to go along and the doctor usually will get a better fix on the problem (This also doesn't cost anything, and the problem may resolve itself spontaneously.) If that relationship and trust isn't present, it's easy for the doctor to simply match the patient with a diagnosis, a CPT Code, perhaps order a test or two, and deliver the indicated treatment. It's also safer from a malpractice standpoint for the doctor to do this, and while this approach may work out OK, a very important element is missing.

Let me explain further. There's something magical about the laying on of hands, about human touch, and I mean this not only in the literal sense but also in the larger context of the patient being "seen" as a person by the doctor. People who enter an examining room and disrobe are often afraid, sometimes very afraid, and the experience of being treated as a fellow human being instead of an object can go a long way towards helping them feel better. There's no CPT Code for treating the patient with respect, for making the patient feel "heard and seen," or for taking the extra time that acknowledges the shared humanity of doctor and patient. I'm not suggesting that there should be such a code, but there's no question in my mind that CPT Codes have helped create an environment in which patients are devalued and diseases have taken center stage. I believe that many people die today in hospitals primarily because they feel that no one really cares about them, not because of their underlying ailment. People who want to get well have a far better chance of getting well; those who lose hope generally don't make it. I can't prove it, but I believe the diseases-rather-than-people mindset has made it more difficult for some patients, especially those with severe illnesses, to maintain hope.

In discussing CPT Codes and their effect on American medicine, I don't mean to suggest that we do away with them. Providers, payers and patients need a method for quantifying the health care that is being delivered, paid for, and received. In our complex and mobile society, the only realistic approach to those needs is some kind of statistical, computer-friendly system – what CPT Codes were originally intended to be. But we cannot lose sight, as I believe American medicine has, of the more important reality that we are treating human beings, not individual collections of five-digit codes. There is no simple solution, but as with most thorny problems, the first step is acknowledging that there is a problem.

Chapter Six

HOW THE HOUSE OF MEDICINE FRAGMENTED AND WHAT THAT MEANS TO PATIENTS

Why We Have Too Many Specialists and Too Few Family Doctors

My oldest son, Tony, is a highly successful orthopedic surgeon, a specialty he chose after a conversation we had while he was still a junior in medical school. Married, planning a family and taking on debt to get his education, Tony needed to decide whether to become a family physician like his father or to specialize in one area of medicine. We were sitting in the living room, just chatting, and he asked me if I had experienced any difference in professional gratification between treating a patient with a sore throat or one with a broken ankle. When I said I hadn't, he declared:

"Well, that's good to hear, because I'm going to become an orthopedic surgeon and I'll make four times as much money as you ever did."

Tony probably makes six times as much money as I ever did. My wife Patty and I didn't raise any dumb kids. But Tony's decision, which I thought then and now made a lot of sense, also is symptomatic of larger forces which have fragmented the House of Medicine to the distinct detriment of patients. The doctor/patient relationship is one of the most significant casualties of this fragmenting, but there are many others, some apparent, some more subtle. As you might by now expect, the primary culprit is money.

Beginning around the time of the development of the CPT Codes I discussed in the previous chapter – and accelerating ever since – the gap between the average incomes of primary care physicians and specialty physicians has widened enormously. Today's medical students, who can easily amass debts of $200,000 completing their schooling, are well aware that established family physicians have average annual incomes of about $150,000 compared with $450,000 and up for specialists.

Not surprisingly, med students are overwhelmingly making the same decision Tony did – choosing a lucrative specialty rather than becoming family doctors. This understandable trend, combined with other forces that have created an exodus of existing family physicians out of medicine, has done enormous damage to what I regard as the nexus of quality health care – the primary care physician. Nationwide, there are now about four specialists for every primary care physician – the inverse of what I consider ideal. What we now have resembles an upended pyramid with a small base of family physicians on the bottom (in every sense) and a large and expanding top portion made up of specialists and sub-specialists. Things are way out of balance, and at some point this structure is likely to tip over.

Before continuing, I want to reiterate that I respect and value specialists. Medicine is far too vast, and advancing far too rapidly, for any one individual to know everything. We have to have medical specialists and they perform a valuable role. But this maldistribution of physicians is having adverse effects on our health care system because each specialty is aggressively pursuing its own narrow interests rather than working for the improvement of the system as a whole. This in part reflects an attitude that can be summarized in the aphorism, "If you're a hammer, every problem becomes a nail." The professional associations of each specialty – be it orthopedic surgeons, rheumatologists, oncologists, radiologists or what have you – focus on issues of concern to their specialty and see the broader questions of health care through that perspective. And since physicians in general feel that their profession is under siege, the human tendency to think of yourself first when in peril also comes into play. "Every man for himself" becomes "Every specialty for itself".

If the fragmentation of the House of Medicine was just a case of the various specialty groups battling over the pie of healthcare dollars, it might be an unfortunate spectacle but not really dangerous. That's not the situation. Fragmentation also has impacted the lives of countless individual patients.

Primary care physicians (I use this term interchangeably with family physicians) once played an invaluable role as both the entry port for health care and the coordinator of the treatment that patients received. This role benefited patients enormously. Because family physicians generally had a history and a relationship with their patients, they could evaluate a specific complaint within the context of the patient's overall health profile – what in more recent years has been characterized as a "holistic" approach. Family physicians who knew their patients could evaluate and prioritize medical issues as they arose, sometimes detecting problems early on when intervention was important (and often less costly), sometimes recognizing that a symptom wasn't really serious and thereby saving the patient from unnecessary anxiety and expense. When treatment was indicated, that care was coordinated and overseen by a physician who knew the patient's overall medical history – what is now called "treating the whole person."

Because primary care physicians are now in such short supply, most patients no longer have a family doctor who can perform these functions. As a result, and CPT Codes have contributed to this, health care has become episodic and disease-oriented instead of holistic. This in turn has contributed to the overuse and misuse of hospital ERs, as well as the growth of Urgent Care and quick-clinic facilities that are the antithesis of treating the whole person.

Episodic care means that patients come in (to the ER, Urgent Care, community health center, quick clinic) with a specific complaint and are treated by a provider (often this is not a physician) who knows nothing about them. Sometimes, if they have insurance and can get approval, they will go directly to a specialist. Either entry point sets both patient and provider almost inevitably onto the road of treating the disease rather than the patient that I discussed in the previous chapter, with all the attendant ramifications. A living, breathing, feeling person becomes a neck, a colon, or a kidney. Because the patient's entry point is the broken leg, stomach ache, rash, or whatever, each problem is treated separately. Believe me here, that approach is a recipe for additional problems.

With episodic care, consistency and coordination of patient treatment become essentially impossible, because the knowledgeable "quarterback" is missing. Each specialty provider is essentially starting with a blank slate and, often worried about malpractice issues, is therefore more likely to practice defensive medicine and order expensive and often superfluous tests. This of course drives up both the cost of the specific encounter and health care expenses overall. Despite this emphasis on defense, episodic care also means an increased likelihood of a provider making a mistake, usually because it's difficult to know with certainty what other medications a patient may be on or what other health issues he or she may have.

Even if they do have a primary care physician who could be coordinating their care, most patients don't get much face time with their doctor. A recent study done at the University of California, San Francisco, found that the average American spends a total of about 30 minutes annually (yes, half an hour a year) with a primary care physician. Patients in this environment sense, correctly, that they are not receiving quality care, and are understandably upset about it. What they are reacting to in large part is the difference between being seen as a person and being seen as a disease. They may or may not articulate it, but they recognize that no one is really looking out for them in the area that matters most – their personal health.

Another place where this fragmentation of medicine has especially sad consequences for patients, and great costs for our society as a whole, is with end-of-life medical care. Because patients are seen as diseases rather than people, the terminally ill are often subjected to needless tests and procedures that make their final days far more unpleasant than they have to be. Futile care is also very costly – more than half of all Medicare expenditures occur for patients during their last 60 days of life. It's impossible to quantify, but some amount of that money did nothing but subject patients to additional misery before they reached the end that awaits us all. A bright spot here is hospice care, which Medicare and private insurers increasingly are covering, and which can provide a "softer landing" for a patient with a terminal illness. Delivered properly, hospice care is both compassionate and cost-effective, bringing patients and their loved ones together to best spend the final days and moments in the closing chapter of the cycle of life.

This is a difficult area, fraught with emotions, denial, malpractice considerations, occasional "miracle" recoveries, and various other issues. Moral hazard (insurance is paying) is also a significant force – we all want to control health care costs in general, but things are very different when that means forgoing care for ourselves or someone we love.

In this environment, the narrow focus of the specialist ("the operation was a success but the patient died") is especially problematic. Trained, conditioned (and compensated) in terms of their particular expertise, they focus on treating the disease. Without a central figure (and the patient is generally in no shape to do this) coordinating and determining what should and shouldn't be done, you get all kinds of egregious behavior. If you've gone through the deaths of your parents and/or grandparents, as I have, you can probably supply your own examples.

The value of a primary care physician in coordinating treatment is perhaps greatest for patients with chronic health care conditions, a group which encompasses many of our elderly (more than 80% of Medicare beneficiaries have at least one chronic condition, about two-thirds have more than one, and 20% have five or more chronic conditions, with this last category accounting for two-thirds of Medicare spending). With the guidance of a family physician, patients with chronic conditions are better able to manage their diseases, obtain care when needed, and connect with support groups. The arrival of the Baby Boomers in the ranks of the elderly guarantees that the number of patients with chronic diseases is going to increase greatly at the same time that the number of primary care physicians is shrinking.

Another reason that family physicians are disappearing is that physicians as a whole are leaving medicine, with the trend most noticeable among older doctors – the group most likely to be primary care physicians. A study done late in 2007 by Merritt Hawkins & Associates, a national physician search and consulting firm, found that half of physicians aged 50 to 65 are frustrated with their practices and plan to sharply cut back or abandon patient care within the next few years. If they follow through on their dissatisfaction, this will have a real impact on health care, because almost half of the physicians in the U.S. are 50 and older. Reimbursement issues, malpractice worries and long hours were the most frequent complaints of the physicians surveyed. The Council on Graduate Medical Education (COGME), a panel of health care authorities, has endorsed a study predicting a shortage of 96,000 physicians by the year 2020.

If you are wondering about the circumstances of primary care physicians in other developed countries, the bottom line is that they are much better. Here's just one example. A 2006 interactive survey done by the Commonwealth Fund/Harris of more than 6,000 primary care physicians in Australia, Canada, Germany, the Netherlands, New Zealand, the United Kingdom, and the United States (including more than 1,000 U.S. physicians) found that our family doctors are struggling in many important areas that directly impact the quality of care. According to the survey, primary care physicians in the U.S. are among the least likely to have extensive clinical information systems or quality-based payment incentives, the least likely to provide access to after-hours care, and the most likely to report that their patients often have difficulty paying for care. Other survey findings:

- Only 28% of the U.S. doctors said they used electronic medical records (EMRs), compared with overwhelming majorities of doctors in the Netherlands (98%), New Zealand (92%), the U.K. (89%), and Australia (79%).
- The U.S. doctors are also the least likely to have systems that provide decision support, such as computerized alerts about potentially harmful drug doses or interactions. Only 23% of U.S. doctors receive computerized alerts; rates elsewhere ranged from 93% (Netherlands) to 40% (Germany).
- At least 40% of U.S. doctors find it "very difficult" or "impossible" to identify patients overdue for a test or preventive care, versus 20% or less in the other countries.
- The U.S. doctors were the least likely to say that their practices allow patients to see a nurse or doctor after regular office hours, without going to an ER or similar facility. Only 40% have such arrangements. By contrast, after-hours care is available in 76% to 95% of the other countries.
- The U.S. doctors were the most likely to report that their patients had difficulty paying for care. Half of the U.S. primary care physicians reported that patients often have difficulty paying for medications, compared with between 7% and 27% in the other countries.

- The U.S. doctors lag well behind their peers in terms of health care information technology. Fewer than 20% of the U.S. primary care physicians reported that their offices supported at least half of 14 IT functions (e.g., automated alerts/reminders, electronic prescribing) cited in the survey. In the other countries, 59% to 83% of doctors reported having such multifunctional capacity.

How did we wind up in a situation where primary care physicians are fleeing medicine, those remaining can't afford to modernize their practices and the income gap between family physician and specialist continues to grow?

A major reason is a shift in attitudes that began with the establishment of Medicare/Medicaid and the CPT Codes that I discussed in the previous chapters. As the fee schedules published by Medicare/Medicaid became the standard reference point for physician reimbursement, the mindset of medicine began to move towards procedures and the specialists who performed them rather than other aspects of treatment such as diagnostic and preventive care. The original values assigned to procedural care were grossly out of proportion to those assigned to the care delivered by family physicians, and this disparity became even greater as time went on.

Several factors drove this increasing divergence. One was the tremendous technological advances that occurred in medicine beginning in the 1960s and accelerating today. Medicine can do things for patients today that were never imagined when the original CPT Codes were developed. As a result, the number of possible procedures has exploded and specialist societies have been able to lobby successfully to maximize the reimbursement for each one.

The overall process by which reimbursement is determined is fairly complex, but like most things run by human beings, it's susceptible to money. Specialists got a head start financially under Medicare/Medicaid and have been able to increase their advantage ever since by influencing the reimbursement process. This takes various forms. If your specialty group is well-heeled, it's easier to fund studies that show the benefits of new procedures in your area of medicine and thereby obtain a CPT Code for them. Once you've got a CPT Code, the game becomes one of lobbying the CPT Editorial Panel I described in the previous chapter and doing other things to move the levers of power. Again, I'm not suggesting malfeasance here – specialists sincerely believe the new procedures will help their patients and very sincerely believe they should be well-compensated for performing them. And because they've got it, they back those beliefs with money. As we all have noticed in other areas of life, the rich tend to get richer.

Specialists also have been aided by the fascination Americans have with medical technology – it's the new surgical procedure or wonder drug that makes headlines, not the everyday diagnostic and preventive care that in fact contributes much more to quality health care as a whole. The combination of more procedures and ever-higher reimbursement rates for them meant that specialists were able to continually leverage technological advances and move further and further ahead of primary care physicians in terms of income. The gap continued to widen and med students – Tony and thousands of others – noticed.

There are other reasons to become a specialist. Generally speaking, specialists also have more mobility in terms of relocating. Family physicians build a practice geographically – serving patients in a particular area. Specialists build a practice based on their expertise in a narrow slice of medicine – patients come to them, often from a considerable distance. If you want to be able to move from one city or area to another, it's a lot easier to do that as a specialist.

Still another factor is that as a society we have come to value the "drama" and "glamour" that surrounds specialists more than the day-to-day treatment provided by family doctors. It's not the pregnancy that's valued, it's the delivery. The family physician who successfully counsels patients at risk for heart disease about diet and exercise will keep many of them from reaching the operating table, but the financial rewards will go to the anesthesiologst who puts them to sleep and the cardiac surgeon who opens them up.

It's also true that a good number of today's medical students have chosen their profession based not on what it will enable them to do for others, but based on what it will do for them. Many of today's med students will acknowledge that they want to work part-time and that being a doctor will enable them to do that. Becoming a specialist furthers this desire to control your life, because you're less likely to be on call and more likely to be doing elective procedures where you can define your hours. Not to pick on any one field, but a simple way to think of this is that dermatologists generally don't get called at midnight or have to work weekends.

It's hard to fault anyone for wanting more control over their life, but this attitude also reflects a shift in priorities – away from the needs of patients and society as a whole in favor of the convenience of the individual physician. In the aggregate, this also has made it more difficult for people to access health care when they need it – specialists are generally more able to work the hours they want instead of those convenient to patients.

This dynamic is also at work in areas you might not expect. Patients who come into a hospital ER suffering from a heart attack generally don't know (or care about) this, but they are quite likely to receive their initial care from a shift-work physician specializing in emergency care. As a shift worker, the ER physician is able to put in his or her hours and then leave business at the office (sometimes the ER physician is part of a group specializing in that type of care, but the effect is the same). Once the patient is stabilized, he or she is then generally transferred to the hospital's cardiac care unit for treatment by a physician who is often on staff at the hospital. Once they're better, they're discharged – to nowhere. They don't have a primary care physician who can help them with the aftermath of their heart attack, and the ER and cardiac specialists who treated them work for the hospital. Because each specialist thinks and acts in terms of their own narrow field of expertise, patients wind up having to fend for themselves once the episode is over. Put this in the category of "I never realized until it happened to me" – and hope to hell that it doesn't.

If patients have family doctors, they can be "handed off" by the particular specialist (I have used a heart attack scenario, but there are many others) and returned to the care of the physician who knows them, knows their history, knows their other problems and can therefore coordinate their aftercare. Handoff issues are a major cause of medical errors and other problems and the reason is fairly simple – in far too many cases, because of the misallocation of physicians we have in this county, there's no one for the specialist or hospital to hand off to.

There are other examples, but the root cause is the mis-allocation of physicians I referenced at the start. It's not hard to see why the physcan community has so many more specialists than primary care physicians – the upended pyramid I referred to earlier – but it's a little more difficult to perceive the consequences of this fragmentation into competing specialties. However, this structure, which devalues personal interaction, preventive medicine, and a holistic approach to treating patients, is a major reason why our health care costs continue to climb even as the overall quality of that care continues to decline. Reversing both trends is going to require a comprehensive reassessment of how we compensate physicians, as well as an impartial reevaluation of the true value that each medical specialty provides. It won't be easy, because these groups are powerful, well-financed, deeply entrenched, and quite conversant with how things really work. But we won't make any meaningful progress on improving the delivery and quality of American health care until and unless physicians move away from a focus on what's good for "me," in this case their specialty, and start thinking and acting on what's good for "we" – our health care system and society as a whole.

Chapter Seven

AN OVERDOSE OF GREED

How Big Pharma Co-opted and Corrupted Legislators, Academic Researchers and Physicians to Create an Incredibly Lucrative Business Model that Has Resulted in an Overmedicated America

Although humans have been consuming various things for various ailments since shortly after the dawn of civilization, no country has ever approached the extremes America has achieved. More than 130 million of us routinely take prescribed medications, according to the U.S. Centers for Disease Control and Prevention, and we buy far more pills per person than any other country. Somewhere between one-third and one-half of the world's pharmaceutical sales occur within the United States.

Over the past 10 years, the number of prescriptions filled in the U.S. has risen by two-thirds and now totals 3.5 billion yearly, according to IMS Health, an authoritative pharmaceutical consulting company. Over the past five years, prescription drug sales have increased by about 11% annually – with prices rising at nearly twice the rate of general inflation – giving the pharmaceutical industry 2008 sales estimated at about $300 billion.

To put that another way, Big Pharma – as the industry is known – is now collecting an average of $1,000 every year from every man, woman and child in the U.S. That's just revenue – pharmaceutical companies also consistently rank near or at the top of all industries in terms of profitability.

As you might infer from these numbers, Americans are overmedicating themselves – and thousands are dying as a result. Our addiction to prescription drugs has caused a very serious problem known medically as polypharmacy, or excessive, unnecessary, or complicating use of multiple medications. This problem is particularly worrisome among the increasing number of older folks. Almost half of all Americans age 65 or older take five or more prescriptions for multiple ailments. One in eight women age 65 or older takes 10 or more medications. Leaving costs aside for a moment, what this sets up is a higher and higher likelihood of adverse drug reactions – one or more medications interacting with another in a way that harms the person's health.

Adverse drug reactions occur for a number of reasons. If a patient has several doctors and they do not coordinate treatment (something increasingly common now that we are driving Primary Care Physicians out of medicine), the physicians may accidentally overload the patient with medications or unknowingly prescribe a harmful combination. A hurried, harried physician may inadvertently prescribe the wrong dosage of a drug – one size does not fit all with drugs because people vary in age, weight, potential allergic reactions, overall health etc. Patients may mix meds and alcohol, may not take their meds as prescribed or, without informing their physician(s), combine them with a non-prescribed "alternative" medication they heard about from a friend or read about on the internet. In the absence of knowledgeable and compassionate oversight, all kinds of things can happen.

You don't need a study to tell you that the more drugs you take, the greater your chances of mixing up a cocktail that will hurt you. But the Veterans Administration has provided some frightening statistics on this subject. Take two different medications and your chances of an adverse drug reaction are about 6%. Take five drugs, and your chances are 50%. Take eight or more drugs and you hit the jackpot – your chances of an adverse drug event are almost 100%. Now think about the one in eight women age 65 or older who takes 10 or more medications – they are playing Russian Roulette – and when the coroner is called, guess what he finds?

"The most common cause of death in our jurisdiction has to do with mixed prescription drug overdoses," says Dr. Jeffrey Jentzen, a medical examiner in Milwaukee and past president of the National Association of Medical Examiners. "They're taking multiple medications that in and of themselves wouldn't prove fatal but in combination do. That's typical around the country."

Some estimates (there are no definitive numbers on this) place the number of annual deaths from adverse drug reactions and mistakes at more than 125,000, which if correct would make pharmaceuticals America's fourth-leading cause of death – after heart disease, cancer and stroke. This is just the headline issue – how many millions of people are slowly destroying their health or functioning poorly because they are essentially poisoning themselves?

Before going any further, I want to stress that there are hundreds of drugs available today that have provided enormous benefits to patients, and to acknowledge that the pharmaceutical industry played a major role, at least initially, in developing them. Millions of lives have been saved, extended and improved by compounds discovered by dedicated researchers and brought to market by drug companies. That's still happening today. However, for reasons I will now lay out, Big Pharma lost whatever moral compass it may once have had and has deliberately transformed itself into a vast money-generating machine whose overriding objective is to maximize sales and perpetuate profits. The industry has persuaded patients, physicians and American society at large that the best response to whatever ails us is usually another pill.

How did this happen? Why are we taking so many drugs and paying so much for them? The short answer is that Big Pharma makes so much money that it has been able to corrupt and ultimately control virtually every step in the process by which drugs are discovered, tested, marketed, and paid for. Big Pharma is also a master at creating "markets" where none existed before.

Looking back on the astonishing transformation of Big Pharma from an OK business to the enormously profitable and hugely influential Goliath it is today, you can't give enough credit to Congress. Time after time, our elected representatives have hand-crafted laws and regulations that either delivered the drug industry obscene profits on a plate or left loopholes large enough for the industry to drive a fleet of bank trucks through. And as Big Pharma accumulated money, it was remarkably ingenious in strategically redeploying this cash in ways that eventually enabled it to control its own destiny. One of the places it recycled a lot of its profits was Washington.

Over time, in bits and pieces, and often unwittingly, our legislators tipped the playing field so sharply in favor of the drug industry that a whole new business model evolved. As a result, Big Pharma doesn't just manufacture medications, it also manufactures the so-called "academic" research that validates the use of those medications and the consumer demand that keeps the prices of prescription drugs ruinously high. Along the way, it also does its best to influence physicians to prescribe highly profitable drugs – often by manipulating and frightening patients into requesting specific medications that are no better than older, less-costly drugs. Big Pharma also uses its financial muscle and lobbying expertise to keep generic drugs off the market for as long as possible and to block attempts to reform the system. As a cartel, and that's what it really is, the pharmaceutical industry is remarkably effective.

In terms of hard evidence demonstrating the clout the drug industry has in Washington, consider the love letter Congress and the White House sent Big Pharma in the form of the Medicare Prescription Drug, Improvement and Modernization Act, which took effect in 2006. Promoted and passed as a way to help seniors with their ever-rising expenses for medications, this legislation essentially handed the drug industry a blank check by expressly prohibiting Medicare from negotiating with drug companies over the prices the government would pay for prescription medications. To put it another way, what our government said was this: Even though other federal agencies (notably the Veterans Administration and the Armed Forces) do negotiate drug prices, Medicare (potentially the biggest buyer of all), may not negotiate prices for the same drugs from the same companies.

Originally projected by the Bush Administration to cost $400 billion over 10 years and sold to a look-the-other-way Congress using that spurious estimate, the tab for this gift to the drug industry was revised shortly after the legislation passed to $530 billion. It is still rising.

I don't think it's necessary to go into much detail here. Excluding one Washington agency from bargaining with its suppliers – while other agencies a few blocks away are bargaining with the same suppliers – speaks volumes as to the influence of the drug industry and the shamelessness with which it operates. The important takeaway is this: your representatives have been bought by Big Pharma, which also has its hooks into the FDA, academia and, I am sad to say, many doctors as well.

To fully comprehend the stranglehold Big Pharma has on our healthcare system, we need to touch briefly on a series of laws that radically changed the drug business. I ask you to stay with me here, because without this background you can't see the true picture of how the drug industry really operates.

1966 – Passage of Medicare and Medicaid

What this landmark legislation did, among other things, was turn on the spigot of government spending for healthcare. Initially, this had little effect on drug prices and the drug industry for the simple reason that there really weren't many medications available at the time. However, the precedent and mechanism for direct government payment for drugs had been put in place. As with other areas of healthcare, private industry now had a pipeline into the federal Treasury that it promptly set about enlarging.

For other reasons, the 1960s and 1970s also saw an increasing emphasis on science and technology that resulted in the discovery and development of many new medications. As we reached the mid-1970s, there were more drugs to buy and government had become a major payer, along with insurance companies.

Patients had also become more accustomed to taking medications. The stage was set.

1980 – Bayh-Dole Act

This bill, enacted at the dawn of the deregulation era ushered in shortly later by Ronald Reagan, fundamentally transformed how drug research is done and what happens to promising new discoveries. Until Bayh-Dole, new medications discovered by universities and small research firms via taxpayer-funded research sponsored by the federal National Institutes of Health were in the public domain, meaning that anyone could work with them. The reasoning was that since the public was paying for the research, the fruits of that effort should be freely available. What Bayh-Dole did was allow those universities and small research firms to patent their discoveries and then license them exclusively to specific drug companies in exchange for royalties. Similar legislation let the NIH itself in on the action, enabling the agency to transfer its discoveries to drug companies. The public was still paying for the research, but now the fruits were going to Big Pharma, which in turn kicked back some of the ensuing riches in the form of royalties paid to researchers, universities and small firms.

I cannot overstate the importance of the shift that occurred because of Bayh-Dole. Money from the profits earned on blockbuster drugs discovered in and around university labs began to flow from Big Pharma to medical schools, their department heads, faculty members and researchers – first a trickle, then a stream and ultimately a river that steadily and relentlessly eroded the ethics of academic research centers and their inhabitants. Small companies, many of them biotech firms, sprang up around universities as professors and researchers realized what was happening and decided to grab a piece of the ever-expanding pie by becoming entrepreneurs. As the great bull market of the 1980s and 1990s wore on, thousands of these small firms went public or were bought by drug giants whose own stock prices had soared. Either way, people who had been stereotypical lab nerds were now driving Porsches and drinking fine wines – and there's something really addictive about that. Once you've savored the high life for a while, you come to believe that you really deserve it.

As I lay out what I believe was a sea change in the attitudes of academia, please bear in mind that I held deanships at three different medical schools. This is what I saw.

Over time, as universities, professors and researchers became accustomed to their newfound chance to get rich, their collective attitudes toward drug companies became more like college cheerleaders than skeptical, show-me researchers working late in the labs. Those in charge of medical schools and teaching hospitals, and those who worked in and around them, had reached the Promised Land and they were not about to turn back. These folks are not stupid, and when they realized that the road to wealth lay in finding new drugs and – very important – in supplying academic stamps of approval to other drugs that Big Pharma was bringing to market, they knew what was expected of them and they complied. As a result, many – and it may even be most – of the studies and research "findings" involving drugs that emanate from some of our nation's most prestigious universities aren't worth a damn.

There are two important takeaways in terms of the consequences of Bayh-Dole: 1) Academic research and academia itself was corrupted and turned into a money game; and 2) Much of the expense of discovering promising (profitable) new drugs, which Big Pharma constantly trumpets as the reason its products cost so much, was shifted – through NIH and associated entities – onto the taxpayer. Big Pharma isn't paying for most of this research – you and I are. Then we pay again, in the form of obscenely high prices for medications the drug industry persuades us we have to have.

1984 – Hatch-Waxman Act

As you know, drugs are sold in two ways – as expensive brand-name medications, which are patent-protected to one company, and as much cheaper generics, which can be manufactured by any company because the patent has expired. Generally speaking, the prices we pay for generics are as close as we're going to come to a "market price" because competition keeps prices down – as it does with other commoditized products. Drugs sold under patent protection, however, are another matter.

While a company holds a patent – and there are several different types of patents – on a product, it can essentially charge whatever it wants for that product. It has a monopoly – the Holy Grail of drug companies. When you combine monopoly pricing with strong and reliable demand – and this demand comes either from patients who really need the drugs (AIDS, cancer, diabetes, etc.) as well as patients who have been manipulated into believing they do (heartburn, most cases of obesity, anxiety, "restless leg syndrome," etc.) – you have, quite literally, a license to steal. This is what makes patents and extending the life of those patents so critically important to drug companies. It's also what makes them so costly. A study in the journal *Health Affairs* estimates that drugs still under patent protection are anywhere from 25% to 40% more expensive in the U.S. than in countries like England, France, and Canada.

Hatch-Waxman was intended to assist generic drug manufacturers and it did so. However, the bill also extended the length of time that brand-name drugs could be protected by patents and in so doing, Hatch-Waxman handed Big Pharma a mechanism the industry would exploit relentlessly.

Patent law is complex, which makes it an ideal playground for the highly paid lawyers of Big Pharma. Multiple patents can be – and routinely are – filed for the same drug, what is sometimes known as "ringing" or "circling" the drug with patents. Additional patents – often for miniscule, essentially irrelevant alterations to the original drug (using a different binding agent is an example) – can be filed during the life of the original patent, the intent being to stretch the life of the company's monopoly as long as possible. Under Hatch-Waxman, a drug that didn't reach market for some time because the FDA was slow (cautious, maybe?) in approving it could have its patent life extended by as much as five years. Hatch-Waxman also enabled Big Pharma to delay the entry of generics in another way. Under the bill, when the maker of a brand-name drug sues the maker of its generic equivalent for patent infringement, a 30-month delay in FDA approval of the generic is *automatically* put in place. In other words, all the brand-name company has to do to get another two-and-a-half years of monopoly protection and pricing, is to claim – not prove – patent infringement.

1992 – Prescription Drug User Fee Act

As the federal body charged with ensuring that the nation's food and drug products are safe, the Food and Drug Administration is an independent agency funded by Congress with taxpayer dollars, right? Well, no. This thrice-renewed (1997, 2002, 2007) legislation authorized pharmaceutical companies to pay fees to the FDA to expedite the approvals of new drugs (seeing the lay of the land, manufacturers of medical devices got a similar deal in 2002). As of 2007, the amount of the fee paid per drug by a company seeking approval for that drug was increased to more than $1 million. In the aggregate, these fees now account for a significant amount of the FDA's overall budget.

You can see what this sets up. In effect, a large number of FDA employees are being paid by the drug companies – and don't think for a moment that they don't understand that. The agency charged with reviewing and approving new drugs and with regulating the industry as a whole gets a significant amount of its funding (about 20% of the overall salaries and expenses of the FDA, 30% within the human drug program and even higher in the approval area) from that industry. Makes you look at your pills in a different light, doesn't it?

While we're on the subject of the FDA, let me pose this question. Since the agency is the nation's guardian of drug safety, the clinical trials that it requires drug companies to conduct in order to win exclusive approval to sell a new drug are pretty tough, right? Well, no. Although neither the FDA nor Big Pharma would ever put it quite this way, all a drug company has to do to get a new drug approved is to demonstrate that it's better than nothing. That's right, better than nothing. Here how that works.

Clinical trials of prospective drugs are not conducted head-to-head against other drugs – either generics or brand-name – already being used to treat a certain condition. These trials are conducted against a placebo – a sugar pill, nothing. Could we set the bar any lower?

Because all they have to beat is a placebo, drug companies can tweak the way a current medication is made, get a patent on the new formulation, put it up against a lowly sugar pill and – voila! – they have a "new" drug that can be marketed under a new name. This is essentially what happened with Claritin and Clarinex, Prilosec and Nexium, Mevacor and Zocor, and dozens of other "copycat" drugs. There's no significant difference between the original and its successor, and the copycat can even be worse than what's already on the market – because the FDA does not require that it be better than an existing medication, only that it be better than a placebo. A clear loophole that Big Pharma drives fleets of bank trucks through.

Once the parameters of this sham really sink in, the real motivations of the drug companies become clear. Another question. If your top priority is profits, what's the best way to obtain them – spend a lot of money researching, developing, testing and bringing a new drug to market, or fiddling around with the formula for a drug you already know has a substantial market so you can "test" it against nothing, get a new FDA-approved pass and start the clock running again? This is why we have so many copycat drugs – it's far cheaper to reformulate an existing medication than it is to develop a new drug.

Again, in fairness I must point out that the overall effectiveness of drugs has improved significantly over the past 30 to 40 years, and the range of conditions that can be addressed with medications has also widened enormously. But at the same time, there are many, many drugs on the market that do essentially the same thing – there is really no discernible benefit to one versus another. There also are many expensive prescription medications that are indistinguishable from their generic counterparts in terms of efficacy. A widely applicable example is drugs for hypertension – high blood pressure. Any honest clinician will tell you that older drugs – those now off patent and available as generics – work just fine, and the drug industry knows this too. But high blood pressure represents an enormous and highly profitable market for Big Pharma. It also has a fear factor that makes it an ideal candidate for direct-to-consumer marketing. As a result, drug companies peddle a number of hypertension medications, skillfully targeting their desired demographic with TV commercials, magazine ads and testimonials from well-known figures whose lives all somehow took a turn for the better when they starting taking (fill in the blank). This is not to say that people shouldn't be concerned about high blood pressure – they should. But there are cheap and effective generics (a simple diuretic is often quite helpful) available to treat hypertension, not to mention the really low cost option of losing weight and exercising.

You can debate whether drug companies are really all that good at finding truly effective new medications – the fact that they outsource much of their R&D and focus largely on finding ways to extend the patent life of profitable drugs would argue otherwise. However, there's one area where Big Pharma must be acknowledged as a world champion: marketing. The industry has been enormously successful at persuading doctors that they should prescribe their products and patients that they should take them. Let's look at how that's done. While we're at it, keep in mind that the costs of marketing drugs are a significant part of their retail prices. In other words, you and I are paying for what I am about to describe.

If I had to single out one behavior on the part of Big Pharma that has done the most harm to the doctor-patient relationship, our collective health and the nation's healthcare system, I would immediately choose direct-to-consumer drug advertising, a practice that is not allowed in almost all other developed countries.

By deploying direct-to-consumer advertising to make an end-run around physicians, the drug industry has demonstrated clearly that what it cares about is profits, not patients. I mean no offense to the person reading this, but unless you have either a medical degree or pharmacological training, you are simply not qualified to judge which cholesterol or hypertension or (pick your malady) drug is best for you, assuming that you need it at all. Whether Joe Athlete or Sally Celebrity or even Dr. Distinguished takes a certain medication has absolutely no bearing on whether it's appropriate for you.

The drug companies know this, but they also know that if a patient asks his or her doctor for a specific brand-name medication it puts the doctor in a very dicey situation. The doctor can 1) spend time educating the patient about different approaches, for which he or she will not be compensated (no CPT Code); 2) try to talk the patient into using another medication, which raises the possibility of a malpractice suit down the road if a problem turns up with that medication (and trust me, that happens); or 3) go along with what the patient wants, realizing that if he/she doesn't, another doctor will. There's no way to quantify how often doctors are choosing option #3, but the ever-increasing volume of prescriptions being written gives us a hint.

In bypassing the physician, who has both medical education and specific knowledge about the person in the exam room, Big Pharma is showing that it cares about neither provider nor patient. The industry is also, albeit unwittingly, telling us what it thinks of its own drugs – they are consumer products to be pushed like toothpaste or deodorant, not medications to be used in a careful, coordinated response to disease.

Direct-to-consumer advertising is intended to put bottom-up pressure on physicians to prescribe specific drugs, often those which Big Pharma knows full well are no better than generics or older, off-patent medications. When these ads say "Ask your doctor about (fill in the blank)," they also send the non-too-subtle message that a doctor who doesn't pull out the prescription pad isn't doing his or her job.

As we all know, you cannot watch television, read a magazine (or medical journal) or ride a bus or subway these days without being subjected to drug advertisements. What you may not realize is this wasn't always the case, and once again the blame lies with those who should be protecting us, in this case the FDA. Until 1997, drug companies could advertise on television only if their commercials listed all of the side effects of a specific drug. Since those side effects usually make for a pretty long list, the practical effect of this rule was to keep most drug ads off TV. However, the FDA relaxed its rule that year, requiring only that drug ads contain those short disclaimers (complete now with serious-looking actors in white coats) you now get at the end of the pitch. The FDA would later tone down its requirements about side effects being listed in drug packaging, meaning that patients now have even less information about what they're taking. One result is unnecessary medication. Another is the overmedication I referenced earlier in this chapter.

So that's one tactic – manufacture bottom-up demand from patients. The second part of the pincer is to "educate" physicians about specific medications and create an atmosphere in which doctors feel comfortable, perhaps even a little obligated, to reach for that prescription pad.

It's important to note here that many of the seminars, lunch lectures and other educational efforts mounted by the drug industry are very valuable to physicians. There are so many medications today that keeping up with all of them is almost impossible. When drug companies sponsor a presentation by an expert in a particular field, they provide the doctors in the audience with information that can and does improve and sometimes save the lives of their patients. When drug companies provide a doctor with free samples, they offer that doctor a way to help poor patients who cannot afford to buy those medications (that's what I usually did with my free samples).

At the same time, there's a line, a point at which the drug companies' educational efforts with physicians becomes something else. Sometimes the line is easy to see, as when a drug company takes a group of doctors and their spouses to a plush resort, all expenses paid, and puts on a couple of two-hour lectures on the mornings of the four-day trip. Sometimes the line is less obvious. If the expert I mentioned above is paid $500 for his presentation, that's one thing. If that expert is paid $100,000 or owns stock in the company that makes the medication he's discussing, that's another. But just where in between those numbers is the line?

Drug companies employ thousands of friendly, generally young and physically attractive representatives known as "detailers" whose job essentially is to make nice with physicians. Though this happens much less than it used to, detailers visit doctors' offices regularly and hand out free drug samples and various other goodies (doughnuts, pens with drug names on them, golf balls, tickets to sports events etc.) Detailers are also found in teaching hospitals, where they are happy to buy a young intern lunch and chat about the latest drug. After all, that intern is going to be prescribing for a long time. Drug companies sometimes pay physicians to allow reps to accompany them as they see patients, supposedly to help the reps learn more about the needs of the physician and his patients. Drug company reps are often present at medical conferences, which leads me to another aspect of doctor cultivation.

Physicians are required, as a condition of license renewal, to stay current on medical information throughout their careers. This is generally accomplished by attending educational events that have been certified as Continuing Medical Education. One national group that certifies such events is the Accreditation Council of Continuing Medical Education (ACCME).

A lecture or seminar or conference may be "worth" three CME units (or some other number), with a physician required to obtain a certain number of CME units each year. In other words, physicians are a captive audience.

Guess who pays for a great many of these events? Yep, it's our friends at Big Pharma. How it's done is this. The accrediting organization, ACCME, contracts with what are known as medical education and communication companies (MECCs) to put on the CME events. So far, so good, but here's the rub: most MECCs are heavily dependent on drug companies for their revenues, raising the question of how objective they are in "educating" physicians.

How objective are MECCs? What are their true motivations? For an answer, here are excerpts from an article in the American Journal of Health-System Pharmacy by Maryam R. Mohassel, a Doctor of Pharmacy who left a career in academia to work for a MECC.

"Most MECCs are for-profit companies whose primary revenue source is the pharmaceutical industry," Mohassel wrote. "MECCs are very forthcoming about their business goals. During its sales pitch to potential clients, one MECC says it 'never loses sight of the strategic value of its programs to enhance its client's corporate image and to strengthen brands.' Another company promotes itself as 'putting the science of medicine to work for you. Preparing and building the market through professional education.'"

In addition to staging CME events for physicians and other medical personnel, MECCs provide another valuable service to Big Pharma. Here's Mohassel again:

"...an employee of a MECC works for clients with a decidedly vested interest in the prescription drug market. I was often reminded of this as a medical writer when I was asked to cast clients' products in a favorable light. This was easy to achieve for novel products with distinct advantages over other agents, but it became a struggle when the assignment involved a "me-too" drug with no apparent additional benefits beyond the competition.

"Then there are the controversies surrounding ghost authorship, which is a service provided by most MECCs. Medical writers ghostwrite scientific articles, yet their act of writing is completely detached from their claim to authorship. When preparing a drug review, the medical writer conducts the literature search, retrieves and reviews the essential articles, organizes the relevant information, and drafts the entire manuscript. The authors listed in the byline are merely prominent clinicians who are paid an honorarium for the insertion of their names. In most cases they do little more than take a last-minute look at the completed manuscript."

In other words, the employees of the MECC write scientific articles about various prescription drugs which are then set forth as evidence of this or that drug's efficacy under the bylines of prominent physicians who are paid for the use of their names. Kind of a different twist on "education," isn't it?

There's another aspect to physician education that is of intense interest to Big Pharma. As we have seen, developing a new drug and bringing it to market to treat a specific condition takes time and money. But what if your drug could be prescribed to treat more than one condition? What if it could be prescribed for several additional ailments, all without the bother of extensive tests and FDA approval? Sound good? Welcome to the wonderful world of "off-label" prescribing.

Physicians can legally prescribe a drug for any use, so if a doctor believes that a medication originally tested and approved for let's say, epilepsy, is also useful for other conditions, let's say insomnia, the physician might also prescribe it for that. What if physicians could be "educated" to believe that this medication is also helpful for patients with migraines, post-traumatic stress disorder, hot flashes, restless legs syndrome – in fact it's almost a cure-all for pain and discomfort? Would you think that the drug would be prescribed more frequently?

You would be right. Let me tell you about Neurontin, which was originally developed in the early 1990s as a treatment for epilepsy by the Parke-Davis division of Warner-Lambert, which later became part of Pfizer. Neurontin had decent sales as an epilepsy drug but it wasn't a blockbuster. So Parke-Davis began "educating" physicians about other uses for Neurontin (remember, a physician can prescribe a drug for any use, not just what's on the label). Parke-Davis sponsored research, hired MECCs to prepare articles on Neurontin and paid academic researchers to put their names on the articles. Parke-Davis sponsored elaborate dinner meetings where the "authors" of the articles would discuss their "findings" about Neurontin with physicians. The authors were paid for their appearances, and Parke-Davis also paid consulting fees to doctors in the audiences. And guess what? Sales of Neurontin began to pick up. In fact, by 2003, Neurontin had sales of some $2.7 billion, most of that for off-label uses. Physician "education" works.

We know all this because in 2004 the drug giant Pfizer, which by then had absorbed Warner-Lambert and Parke-Davis, settled a whistleblower suit that described what was going on in some detail. Pfizer pleaded guilty to illegal marketing and paid $430 million to settle criminal and civil charges that had arisen in connection with Neurontin.

Because they can affect prescribing patterns and volumes for both approved and off-label uses of various medications, well-known physicians who can influence other physicians are a prime target of the drug industry, which lavishes a lot of money on them in the form of "consulting fees." Consider the case of Dr. Charles B. Nemeroff, a prominent psychiatrist at Emory University who, according to press reports, earned $2.8 million in fees between 2000 and 2007 and at one point apparently was consulting for more than 20 drug and device companies at the same time. Busy man.

One of the drug companies that paid Dr. Nemeroff is Glaxo, which makes the anti-depressants Paxil and Wellbutrin. Here are some of the places where he spoke at educational conferences attended by physicians: the Hyatt Key West Resort in Key West, FL; the Bacara Resort & Spa in Santa Barbara, CA; the Four Seasons Resort in Jackson Hole, WY. Education? Maybe so. Luxury and fun? You bet. Were there some friendly drug company reps chatting up doctors at those conferences? Good bet.

It's a tad unfair to single out Dr. Nemeroff, because he is not alone in these arrangements. Prominent physicians from Harvard, Stanford and many other universities have been on the payroll of Big Pharma for years (see chapter on medical schools). The problem is, we have no comprehensive way of determining who's getting how much from which companies, and for what.

Some states do keep track of payments from drug companies to those working in health care, and here's what their records show. Between 1997, when Minnesota began its database, and 2005, drug companies made at least $57 million worth of payments to more than 5,500 doctors, nurses and other health care workers in the state. More than 20% of Minnesota's licensed physicians took money from drug makers. In Vermont, for the 12 months covering July 2005 to June 2006, 81 drug manufacturers spent a total of $2.25 million on "fees, travel expenses, and other direct payments to Vermont physicians, hospitals, universities and others for the purpose of marketing their products," the state reported.

Physicians are often indignant and even outraged when these matters are raised, insisting that they can't be bought with free lunches and golf shirts. I have been in medicine for more than 40 years and I never once prescribed or recommended a drug based on anything else except what was best for the patient. Many of my colleagues are the same way. Unfortunately, there are plenty who aren't. Parke-Davis tracked the prescribing patterns of physicians who were hired to discuss the drug and who attended the dinner meetings and found a reported 70% increase in prescriptions for Neurontin. Big Pharma doesn't do this because it doesn't work.

Physicians do need to stay current on advances in drug therapies. They need to be able to listen to and learn from and ask questions of experts who specialize in, say, diabetes. As patients, we want our doctors to be knowledgeable and there's no particular reason why physicians shouldn't be able to obtain that knowledge in a nice setting. Most doctors work very hard, and there's nothing inherently wrong with mixing business and pleasure. At the same time, there's no doubt as to what the drug companies are trying to accomplish in courting physicians – they're trying to sell their most profitable products. The question of when legitimate education strays over the line into something more closely resembling bribery is more difficult than it may seem. However, like Supreme Court Justice Potter Stewart's famous definition of pornography, we know it when we see it.

It's important at this juncture to reflect on who owns the drug companies and what their motivations are. The bottom line is this: drug companies are primarily owned by – and beholden to – Wall Street firms such as hedge funds, mutual funds, banks, insurance companies, pension fund managers and the like. These are not charitable institutions – they are interested in seeing profits. Wall Street institutions own 69% of Pfizer, the world's biggest pharmaceutical company. They own 73% of Merck, 65% of Johnson & Johnson, 68% of Abbott Labs, 73% of Bristol-Myers Squibb, and similar percentages of other major drug makers. Wall Street owns Big Pharma, and they work together.

Partially because of who owns them, partially because higher profits generally means higher stock prices (which in turn means the executives' stock options are worth more), and partially because of how they have evolved, drug companies don't really conceptualize what they do as helping patients. Oh, they'll bombard us with warm and fuzzy commercials showing a sweet little lady whose arthritis is better because of Celebrex, but that's not how they really think. They don't see people, they see "markets." This is why they focus on "blockbuster" drugs and why they go to such lengths to protect their patented, brand-name, expensive medications.

Here's an example on how drug companies will fight to protect their brand names. The world's best-selling drug (and our nation's most widely prescribed medication) is Pfizer's Lipitor, a cholesterol-lowering agent which has made enormous amounts of money for the company. Lipitor and other cholesterol-lowering drugs belong to a class of drugs called statins which are the biggest pharmaceutical "market," accounting for spending of more than $20 billion annually in the U.S. alone.

Statins have been around for a while and thus have been researched quite thoroughly, which makes head-to-head comparisons with generics easier. Lipitor, which is protected by a ring of patents that expire in 2010, is not available as a generic. However, a very similar drug made by Merck, Zocor, lost its patent protection in 2006 and a generic version of Zocor called simvastatin is now widely available. Simvastin is much cheaper than Lipitor. Depending on where and how you buy it, Lipitor costs about $2.50 to $3 a day. Simvastin, by contrast, costs between 75 cents to $1 a day at most retail pharmacies and as little as 10 cents a day at discount pharmacies.

Big difference. Insurance companies (which are also about making money) have pushed doctors and patients to switch to simvastin, which would mean lower costs for the insurance companies and lower sales and profits for Pfizer.

What to do? Well, Pfizer mounted a huge campaign to protect Lipitor that included TV and magazine ads, intense lobbying in Washington, and – here are the fear tactics – promotion of a study concluding that British patients who switched to simvastatin had more heart attacks and deaths than those who remained on Lipitor. Sounds ominous, doesn't it? Would you risk a heart attack to save a couple dollars a day?

There's a problem with this line of attack, though. Guess who did the British study? You bet – it was Pfizer itself. And here's another surprise – the company's hard-working, dedicated researchers came up with a study that "...will run counter to everything that's been published to date if it's true," according to Dr. Thomas H. Lee Jr., a prominent cardiologist who is president of a network of about 5,000 doctors in Partners HealthCare, the health system formed by Massachusetts General Hospital and Brigham and Women's Hospital in Boston.

"Simvastatin is much less expensive to society over all and to patients," Dr. Lee told the media. "If you put patients on generics, the chances that they're taking their medications six months later are higher than on a brand name drug. I think that a few hundred dollars a year does matter."

Pfizer also took other actions to protect Lipitor. Generic Lipitor is made by an Indian company called Ranbaxy Laboratories Ltd., which has challenged Pfizer's patents on the blockbuster drug. Wall Street was concerned that if Ranbaxy prevailed, it would be able to start selling generic Lipitor in the U.S. around the middle of 2010. Good for patients, as Dr. Lee points out, but not good for Pfizer's profits. So Pfizer and Ranbaxy made a deal. Ranbaxy agreed to wait until Nov. 30, 2011 to start selling its generic Lipitor in the U.S., and Pfizer agreed to drop efforts to block Ranbaxy from selling the generic when Lipitor patents expired in various other countries around the world. This included important markets such as Canada, Belgium, the

Netherlands, Germany, Sweden, Italy and Australia. They carved up the world "market."

So Pfizer got more time to sell the higher-priced Lipitor to U.S. patients, and Wall Street was pleased. Here's how Mike Krensavage, principal of Krensavage Asset Management LLC, described the situation to Reuters:

"Pfizer is a more attractive company today because this deal would delay Lipitor generics from five to 20 months, and spare Pfizer $3 billon to $11.7 billion in lost Lipitor sales over that period."

Here's how Standard & Poor's described that deal in its assessment of the prospects for Pfizer's stock:

"PFE recently reached an agreement with generic drugmaker Ranbaxy delaying that company's U.S. launch of a generic version of Lipitor until the end of November 2011. We had been expecting generics in the first half of 2010. We believe this deal adds cash flow and eases near-term dividend jitters (for Pfizer)."

Here's how Ranbaxy Chief Executive Malvinder Singh summed things up, again to Reuters:

"It was best to bring certainty for both organizations. The biggest part for us is in the United States where we will launch with certainty and without any risk."

Did you hear any mention of patients in those statements? Me neither.

In fairness, these companies, and the others that comprise Big Pharma, are simply doing what they are set up to do – make money. If we were talking about selling shoes, or hair spray, or vacuum cleaners, or various other discretionary items, all the deal-making and dueling studies and advertising and lobbying might be acceptable tactics in a free and open marketplace. But as I've pointed out previously, that's not what we're talking about. Healthcare is not a free market.

When you have senior citizens skipping meals and cutting their meds in half to compensate for the costs of drugs that now account for roughly one in every five dollars spent on healthcare, this kind of behavior is not just unacceptable, it's reprehensible.

I think you get the picture. Big Pharma's incredibly lucrative business model, assembled with the repeated help of our legislators, is roughly as follows:

- Offload much of the research and development costs of developing your product onto the taxpayer.
- Manipulate patent laws and the FDA to obtain monopoly pricing on your product. Use those same patent laws and various other means to prevent generics from under-pricing your expensive prescription products.
- Set things up so that the academic researchers evaluating your product stand to profit personally from favorable reviews.
- Generate demand using those favorable reviews and an immense marketing budget to appeal directly to consumers and to persuade physicians to prescribe your product.
- Use the money you make to influence legislators and get laws passed that maintain your monopoly position. (Big Pharma's lobbying machine is Washington's biggest, and includes former government officials and legislators who know how to get things done).
- Sit back and enjoy – you've got products that 1) people really need, or 2) you've manipulated people into believing they really need, and you can pretty much charge what you want.

If you really take it apart, the dynamics of the drug business work like this. The useful medications the industry sells to folks who truly need them give Big Pharma cover to exploit patients, physicians and payers by selling other drugs of dubious value at inflated prices. The value – and it is real – represented by medications that genuinely help people gives Big Pharma a formidable weapon that it does not hesitate to wave about. Tighten regulations, level the playing field with more competition, crack down on outrageous profits and the consequence, we are told, will be that desperately ill patients won't be able to get the medications they need. What's more, promising new drugs won't be developed. This is essentially medical blackmail – let us gouge you or you won't get the medications you need.

There's another culprit here, and it's us. As a society, we've come to believe – even demand – that we feel good all the time. Big Pharma has played a role in fostering this attitude, but it didn't create it. Faced with a choice of lowering our blood pressure through diet and exercise or medication (insurance is paying, after all), far too many of us reach for the pill bottle. When we get sad or depressed or anxious, which is part and parcel of being alive, we want instant chemical relief. We don't want to grow old and frail, we want four-hour erections into our '80s. We want, we want, we want. This is an environment made to order for Big Pharma, and the drug companies are experts at exploiting it. They're not forcing these pills down our throats – we're taking them.

This is a complex issue. As I've said, the medications discovered in the past 40 years have been enormously beneficial to millions of people – and it takes money to fund the research that found those valuable medications and will find more. There's nothing inherently wrong with publicly owned companies making a profit – that's what their shareholders expect them to do. Impartial and credible medical experts should be paid to share their knowledge with physicians who want to stay current on the latest drug therapies so they can help their patients.

At the same time, there's no question that the drug business has gone badly astray. It's about profits, not patients, and that's simply wrong. We're not talking about toothpaste here, we're talking about people's health, about their very lives.

We need to re-examine and reform the whole way in which new drugs are discovered, developed and patented. We need to restructure the FDA. We need more transparency in terms of how drugs are marketed, including an overhaul of the Continuing Medical Education process. Patients need to know – and doctors need to be willing to disclose – whether their physicians are being paid by the drug industry and if so, how much and for what. We need to think about what happens when medications – and this is true of medical devices, hospital care and various other forms of healthcare – are delivered by publicly-held, for-profit corporations whose major owners are Wall Street institutions. We need – each of us individually – to think critically about whether we really need that pill and about the long-term consequences of what we're ingesting.

Ultimately, you can't legislate ethics, or morality, or responsibility. Trying to do so provides lobbyists with a handsome living, sets up a cat-and-mouse loophole game, and perpetuates the broken system we have now. We need a bottom-up reboot of Big Pharma that reverses its current priorities, and that can only come from the collective power of patients.

Chapter Eight

DAMAGED IN MEDICAL SCHOOL

How Specialist Physicians, Elitist Thinking, and an Emphasis on Money Dominate Our Nation's Medical Schools and Warp the Values of Medical Students

Why does someone choose to become a doctor? Contrary to some popular stereotypes, it's not about money, at least not at first. There are many, many easier ways to make money, and much more of it. Having been a dean at three medical schools and put five kids through medical school, I have been around a great many med students. Based on what I have observed first-hand over the years, I can assure you that most of the young men and women who choose careers in medicine genuinely want to help and heal.

So what happens to them? What transforms these earnest young people, all of whom are bright and hard-working, into the impatient, impersonal, money-oriented physicians so many of us have encountered time and again? A lot of things happen, some of which I have already discussed. But one of the major character-deforming experiences is med school itself.

Like many of our other institutions, America's medical schools have been transformed by the over-riding emphasis on money and power and prestige that has characterized our society as a whole in the last few decades. This is particularly unfortunate, because med schools play a major role in shaping the values and attitudes of the young men and women who spend several intense years at these educational institutions beginning to learn what it really means to be a doctor. Med school also is where students make choices that will determine what type of medicine they practice, which in turn influences what benefit they will be to society as a whole.

Our med schools generally produce physicians who are well informed on the latest medical advances and are technically quite proficient at running tests, performing various procedures, prescribing medications and so on. Where these new physicians are woefully deficient is an area that is difficult to measure but really much more important – how they regard and behave toward the living, breathing, often-time frightened human beings who come to them for help. The foundational principles that guided most physicians just a few decades ago are not being passed on to our newest doctors, and we're all suffering as a result.

As I lay this out, bear in mind that we're talking here about young men and women whose ethical and moral value systems are still being formed. They're still kids, really, and the role models they encounter during med school and the three-to-five-year residencies that follow it are tremendously influential in shaping the attitudes, values and behaviors they will later display in dealing with patients and the world in general. Let's look at who and what they encounter, and as we do, please remember that I'm not theorizing – I rubbed shoulders with the people I'm about to describe for many, many years.

It's important to understand that the physician-professors who exert such a great influence on our med students have themselves been enormously influenced by the vast streams of money our academic research centers have attracted in recent years. Dollars are sloshing all around these faculty members and over time they come to believe – sincerely, I think – that they are entitled to take home a disproportionate share of them. We've seen the same tone-deaf mentality on Wall Street recently among executives who are really convinced that their yearend bonuses should be in the millions of dollars regardless of what kind of shape their companies (and the shareholders) are in.

Although there are great disparities among physician incomes, because of how our health care reimbursement system is set up, doctors who choose to practice medicine in a certain way can make a great deal of money. What happens in med school is that students overwhelmingly encounter physician-professors who have made the money choice and who need to justify it. Consciously and unconsciously, these faculty members inculcate students with their values – and this contributes to the impersonal treatment many patients encounter from newly-minted physicians today. In some respects, it's not the students' fault. Not only are they influenced by the role models they encounter, they are admitted in the first place based on criteria that emphasize test scores, scientific aptitude, an orientation towards research – all factors that serves the needs of the faculty rather than the needs of society. The med school admission process has become a self-aggrandizing exercise rather than a mechanism for selecting prospective physicians who will serve the needs of society. Medicine is a team sport, not an individual exercise. Collaborative ability, openness to other ideas and possibilities, true connection with patients – these attributes are hard to measure but absolutely essential in a good physician.

Why does someone choose to become a doctor? Often, it's because of the example set by a parent – many med school students are the children of physicians. But because the human qualities I have cited are no longer valued as much as test scores, physician-parents who have these qualities are less likely today to encourage their children to go into medicine. Again, I speak from experience. Like most parents and grandparents, I compare notes with my professional colleagues as to what careers they are encouraging their children and grandchildren to pursue. What I have noticed is that if the physician is empathetic and chose medicine as a way to serve humanity, he or she is less likely to recommend that career to the new generation. When, on the other hand, I chat with physician-parents I know to be technically quite proficient but short on empathy, they often have urged their children to follow in their footsteps. This admittedly unscientific survey tells me we are going in the wrong direction.

For better or for worse, I did encourage my children (and now my grandchildren) to go into medicine. Let's look at what they have encountered.

My youngest son, also named Sam, went to the University of Southern California Medical School while I was Senior Associate Dean there. Like all med students, Sam went on rounds at County-USC Hospital with various physician faculty members. These physician-professors usually take a group of med students to see patients, commenting on the patients' specific conditions along the way and lecturing their young charges on a variety of matters pertaining to the overall practice of medicine.

One day Sam went on rounds with a distinguished physician who was the head of the school's general internal medicine department, but more importantly, also the head of the ethics department. As he was shepherding the dutiful young residents around, this doctor told them that they should try to delay discharging patients for as long as possible because "that's what keeps the beds full."

That's about as clear a declaration of values as you're going to get – keeping the beds full means more money for the hospital, albeit at the expense of some other party. It also ignores the best interests of the patient. Keeping people in longer than necessary means subjecting them to more of what very few regard as a pleasant experience, as well as exposing them to all the dangers present in any hospital.

In addition to warped values, this anecdote also illustrates the enormous arrogance that is all too prevalent among med school faculty physicians, most of whom regard themselves as an ultra-elite class whose decisions and actions are not to be questioned. This is a key point – it's not just the actions and decisions and rationalizations of med school faculty and administrators that are the problem, though many of those are reprehensible enough. The larger issue, at least in terms of what happens to impressionable young med students, is the entitlement mindset these role models exhibit, a mindset that says it's OK for them to game the system, treat patients as pawns, act in their own self-interest, essentially to do whatever they want because of who they are.

Recently, some of the value judgments and ethical attitudes at our most prestigious medical schools have begun to be questioned, and what's turning up isn't pretty. Sen. Charles E. Grassley, an Iowa Republican, has been looking into payments by pharmaceutical companies to physicians on the faculties at universities such as Harvard and Stanford. Grassley's office identified two prominent Harvard psychiatrists, Dr. Joseph Biederman and Dr. Timothy Wilens, who, according to media reports, apparently each under-reported earnings of more than $1.6 million apiece from drug makers, possibly in violation of federal and university rules. Grassley also questioned the judgment of Dr. Alan Schatzberg, chairman of Stanford University's psychiatry department, who Grassley said controlled more than $6 million worth of stock in a company called Corcept Therapies, a company he co-founded. Dr. Schatzberg also was the principal investigator on a study funded by a National Institute of Mental Health (NIMH) grant into the efficacy of a drug Corcept was developing.

Was it a conflict of interest to control a hefty chunk of stock in a company while taking government money to investigate whether that company's product was beneficial? Stanford apparently saw nothing wrong with that arrangement (perhaps because it is not uncommon in academia) until Grassley began to poke around, after which the university 1) sold it own stock in Corcept and 2) temporarily replaced Dr. Schatzberg as the lead investigator on the NIMH grant "to eliminate any misunderstanding."

In what has become a potential embarrassment for one of our nation's most prestigious institutions, a student in a first-year pharmacology class at Harvard Medical School decided to check into the background of a professor who seemed intent on trumpeting the benefits of cholesterol drugs while minimizing their potential side effects. His online investigations revealed that the professor, a full-time faculty member at Harvard Med, was also collecting consulting fees from

10 drug companies, including five which manufactured cholesterol drugs.

Whether or not that was improper is a matter of intense debate at Harvard, but it's interesting that the professor didn't disclose his drug company connections to his students. Then again, maybe not. After the students pushed for – and won – a university requirement that all professors and lecturers disclose their industry ties, one Harvard professor was forced to disclose 47 company affiliations. Many others had multiple fee arrangement with medical companies. The disclosure rules also turned up the information that about 1,600 of 8,900 professors and lecturers had (or a family member had) a financial interest in a business related to their teaching, research or clinical care.

In a case of turnabout, the American Medical Student Association, a national group that rates how well medical schools monitor and control drug industry money, gave Harvard an "F" grade. Yale got a "C," with a "B" going to Stanford, Columbia and New York University. The University of Pennsylvania got an "A."

Here's a comment from David Tian, 24, a first-year Harvard Medical student, as quoted in The New York Times on March 2, 2009: "Before coming here, I had no idea how much influence companies had on medical education. And it's something that's purposely meant to be under the table, providing information under the guise of education when that information is also presented for marketing purposes."

These are not isolated examples. A study whose findings were reported in the Journal of the American Medical Association (JAMA) in 2003 concluded that roughly two-thirds of academic research centers (our most respected and prestigious med schools) own stock in companies that sponsor research at those same research centers. A 2007 study published in JAMA focusing on the chairs of med school departments found that two-thirds received departmental income from pharmaceutical companies and three-fifths took money personally.

Don't med schools have policies dealing with potential conflict-of-interest situations? Well, they're getting around to it. In June 2008, after several years of embarrassing disclosures regarding drug company payments to faculty physicians, the Association of American Medical Colleges (AAMC) issued a set of suggested guidelines on conflicts of interest. Some med schools are adopting these guidelines, or variations of them, and some aren't – there's nothing binding about the AAMC recommendations. And you have to wonder why med schools are just recently adopting conflict-of-interest policies, and whether it's only because they've been embarrassed into it.

In many ways, this is the heart of the problem. While it may be a step forward that med schools are adopting conflict of interest policies, it raises a larger question. Shouldn't concepts like integrity, putting patients before profits, and accepting that being a physician entails personal sacrifice be the foundational principles that students learn and med schools practice? To put it another way, why does a university have to spell out for faculty members that there's a problem with having a substantial financial interest in a company while managing a research study into whether that company's product is beneficial? Why does a university have to force its professors to tell their students that they are being paid by the companies whose products they are discussing in class?

I think we know the answer. The ubiquity of practices like those I have cited is a telling sign of the absence of ethics at our med schools. Instead of being positive role models, the universities, their department chairs and their faculty are instead sending the message that it's OK to get whatever you can from wherever you can. They're also sending another message, one which permeates every corner and level of health care, namely that what matters is money, not patients or making a contribution to societal needs. This is the attitude the doctor that Sam followed on rounds was exhibiting.

They are probably the most blatant item, but drug company payments are only part of the financial value system at med schools. Other dynamics include the fierce competition for government research grants, the horrendous increases in med school tuition, and the inflated incomes of tenure-protected professors and deans.

Let's look at tuition, because there's an important ripple effect in terms of the behavior and choices of med school graduates. There are about 125 med schools in the United States, with more planned. These schools receive applications from about 42,000 students each year and admit about 18,000. In other words, the demand for slots is at least twice the supply.

According to the AAMC, tuition and fees at med schools have been increasing 11.1% annually in recent years. I don't know too many businesses – and make no mistake, that's what med schools have become – that have been able to increase prices like that year after year. I do know that doctors' incomes have not been rising at anywhere near that rate. Why have med schools raised their tuition and fees so sharply? Because they can – supply and demand. As a side note, med school tuition increases are part of a larger trend. The National Center for Public Policy and Higher Education recently reported that published college tuition and fees rose by 439% between 1982 and 2007, adjusted for inflation, while median family income for the same period increased just 147%. What this means is that that most students arrive at med school already in debt and then go under even further. Let's see how far.

In 2006, sharply rising tuition/fees saddled med school graduates with a median debt of $120,000 for those getting their diplomas from public universities and $160,000 for those graduating from private universities. Almost all students then defer payment on their debts during their three-year residencies, by which times these figures will have grown to about $150,000 and $200,000 respectively. These are median numbers (half of the students will have lower debt loads and half will have higher) and, in my experience, tend to understate the realities. What I can say with complete assurance is that it's not uncommon at all for those completing their residencies to have debt loads of $250,000 and more. How's that for pressure?

At this point, a newly minted doctor is usually pushing 30 and often has a spouse and a couple of kids. He or she now has to make an enormously important decision, one that will affect all of their lives, which is where to locate and begin to practice medicine. Remember, although they are fairly sophisticated by now in terms of medical knowledge, the majority of these fresh physicians have never spent much time at all in the "real world." So how do they make that momentous decision? Most go to the default value system that has been front, center and supreme during their years in med school – they make a decision based on money. New physicians tend to locate in areas where reimbursement rates and income are high, because that's where they can make the most money. One result of this mindset is that our rural areas are desperately short of physicians.

These debt loads also play a major role when students decide what kind of medicine they're going to practice. Well before the third year of med school, which is when students have to decide what area of medicine they're going to specialize in, they do some simple math. If they choose to become a primary care physician (PCP), they will make far less both immediately and over the course of their careers than if they choose to specialize in one particular area of medicine. Not surprisingly, the vast majority choose a specialty where they will perform a high volume of procedures – again based on the values that have been exhibited by their role models, most of whom are specialists or sub-specialists.

In discussing the dilemma of rising educational debt levels that are far outstripping income gains for physicians, the same AAMC study, aptly titled *Medical School Tuition and Young Physician Indebtedness*, puts it succinctly:

"These trends indicate eventual hardship for both primary care doctors and specialists, but the absolute value of compensation is much higher for specialists. In comparison with our base year 2006 figure of $216,600 for all physicians, primary care physicians probably earn 30% less, and the typical specialist earns 16% more. The threshold for repayment pain will thus be reached much sooner for primary care physicians than for specialists."

Run those numbers, and you'll wind up with an average income of about $150,000 for primary care physicians and $250,000 for specialists. In reality, the disparity is far greater than that – the rule of thumb in the medical community is that specialists earn two to three times as much as primary care physicians. For sub-specialists in a field that is heavily procedure-oriented the ratio can get up to 10-to-one. Remember, in our health care system doctors get paid based on how many procedures they do.

Today's med students understand this, and are also well aware of the monetary realities. This awareness is occurring earlier and earlier – students on premed tracks in college can tell you what a hand surgeon makes. But if they don't enter med school with a predisposition to become specialists, they acquire it rapidly. Primary care, also referred to as family medicine, is regarded as kind of dull by med school professors, most of whom are specialists and sub-specialists. They let students know that in their view family medicine simply isn't glamorous or exciting in the way that being a cardiac surgeon or neurosurgeon or kidney transplant specialist is. This devaluation of the societal contribution made by primary care physicians has become so pervasive that only a handful of med schools now offer credible and comprehensive training in family medicine. As a result, we're facing a critical shortage of new primary care physicians – and the older generation of family doctors is retiring or simply giving up on practicing medicine.

I've mentioned the importance of role models in influencing the moral and ethical standards that med students develop. In this regard, let's look quickly at the physician-professors who populate the faculties of our med schools.

Med school professors come in two flavors – academics whose orientation is supposedly research and clinical professors whose orientation in today's health care system is on performing procedures. At one time, both types were essentially university employees but this is no longer true.

As I have explained elsewhere, today's research professors are quite likely to have founded or have stakes in companies where they can leverage their academic findings. This poses some obvious questions. Who are these folks really working for? What is their overriding motivation? Are they primarily interested in educating the next generation of physicians, or are they using their positions as faculty members to develop outside revenue sources to supplement their already exorbitant salaries? What is the ethical climate in medical school when two-thirds of the chairs receive departmental income from pharmaceutical companies and three-fifths take money personally (the findings of the 2007 study published in JAMA)?

There's nothing inherently wrong with a research professor setting up a company and participating in some of the rewards associated with his or her research. I'm not suggesting that physician-professors take a vow of poverty. But bear in mind that the funding for most medical research essentially comes from the taxpayers. In other words, when Professor Jones capitalizes on his research findings by founding a company, he's doing so based on discoveries made with seed money that came largely from you and me. That's not quite the same as Bill Gates or Steve Jobs or William Packard tinkering with computer codes or electronic parts in their garages and later turning their efforts into Microsoft or Apple or Hewlett-Packard.

The financial route for clinical professors is somewhat different but the destination is the same. At one time, clinical professors also were primarily university employees. They treated patients in county or city hospitals, but drew their paychecks from their universities. However, as the revenue streams provided by Medicare and Medicaid grew over the years, this changed. Clinical professors treated patients in hospitals affiliated with their universities and billed Medicare and Medicaid for reimbursement. Like their research-oriented colleagues, they now had other sources of income. In fact, universities facilitated this, setting up practice plans (essentially mechanisms for professors to treat patients and be reimbursed) for their faculty. In time, this expanded to include payments by private insurers as well, so today's clinical professor is getting a paycheck from his or her med schools and also being reimbursed by Medicare, Medicaid and private insurers for treating patients.

There's nothing inherently wrong with this either. Professor-physicians, almost all of them specialists, hone their skills and patients – many of whom are poor and might otherwise have trouble obtaining care – are treated by some very capable doctors. But there's another effect too, one that med schools don't like to acknowledge. As I have explained elsewhere, the income of specialists depends on how many procedures they perform. This is especially true for Medicare and Medicaid patients, where the amounts reimbursed for this or that procedure are generally less than what the doctor can get from a private insurer. So again, the name of the game – and remember, students are taking this all in – becomes volume. How many procedures can we bill? Keep those beds full!

In addition to this monetary orientation, research-oriented professors focused on capitalizing on their individual specialties and clinical professors intent on performing as many procedures as possible are also signs of something else – an enormous shift in the way medicine as a whole is conceptualized.

We tend to think of medicine as an ancient art, and indeed it is. But until the 1940s, when penicillin came into use, physicians really couldn't do all that much for their patients. In fact, many of the treatments of the 19th and early 20th centuries may have done more harm than good. The development of modern medicine, which encompasses such major strides as antibiotics, organ transplantation, childhood vaccines, anti-inflammatory and anti-psychotic drugs, enormously improved diagnostic and imaging capabilities – just to name some of the advances – is a relatively recent phenomenon. We are now doing procedures and administering treatments that would have stunned my professors. We have advanced so far so fast – and this pace is accelerating – that we have overwhelmed any individual physician's ability to fully understand his or her specific discipline. You won't hear many doctors acknowledging that, but it's true. This in turn has led to the establishment of many sub-specialties – ever narrower fields of discipline where the practitioners treat exotic ailments and extract whopping fees in return.

These sub-specialists congregate at med schools that are also academic research and referral centers – places where patients wind up when nobody else can solve their particular problem. While it's beneficial for med students to be exposed to these subspecialties and their practitioners, it also reinforces the message that the real money is in knowing as much as you possibly can about a specific organ or disease. The value of empathy, of seeing and caring for the living, breathing, often-times frightened person in front of you, is just not part of the equation. This is the shift in the conceptualization of medicine that I'm talking about, and it's profoundly important.

We need specialist physicians, both as a society and as individuals, but we first need to keep in mind that we're treating people, not organs or joints. When a patient has an issue so complex or rare that a primary care physician cannot deal with it, we need to be able to bring more specialized expertise to bear on the problem. But that's not what we're doing. We're pushing med students into becoming specialists – for all the reasons I have delineated – and then we're pushing patients into seeing them far earlier and more often than is warranted. On the patient side, we have our society's worship of technology, the fact that somebody else is paying, and the belief that more is always better, among other factors. On the physician side, we have the considerations I have mentioned and the fact that our med schools are turning out new doctors with immense debt loads and value systems that emphasize personal gain.

In many ways, what has happened in our med schools mirrors what has happened in the corporate world. These specialists and sub-specialists make enormous amounts of money, and over time they develop correspondingly enormous senses of entitlement. In their minds, rules, regulations, ethics, even commonsense notions of what's right and wrong somehow just don't apply to them. Of course, the fact that they have tenure encourages this. The same is true, to varying degrees, with most of their colleagues and the administrators who preside over these business enterprises called medical schools.

The truth is that our med schools are charging students more than is warranted and thus burdening them with huge debt loads when they begin to practice. They are also exposing them to role models who emphasize lucrative and episodic medical specialties rather than health care provided to a person over time, and infusing them with an arrogant amorality that views the value system of paychecks over patients as the way things ought to be. Once you get past being awed by the ivy-covered columns and patrician attitudes of the professors and deans, you can see today's med schools for what they really are – highly profitable, bottom-line oriented businesses that are launching pads to higher incomes for their graduates.

Lest you think that I am alone in my views, let me quote from a recent report entitled "Revisiting the Medical School Educational Mission at a Time of Expansion" which grew out of a 2008 medical education summit sponsored by the Josiah Macy, Jr. Foundation and chaired by Jordan Cohen, M.D., a former president of the AAMC. The summit brought together medical and institutional leaders from throughout the country who were critical of what they described as the "conspicuous gap that exists between the rhetorical commitment to high professional standards and the actual behavior on display in many present-day learning environments." The panelists also cited what they termed an "ethical imperative" to relieve the financial burden that med school graduates incur, which they said may discourage graduates from choosing "less lucrative but potentially more socially responsible career paths."

In the final analysis, med schools are societal institutions with three primary obligations – to conduct academic research that advances our overall knowledge of medicine, to educate and train new doctors, and to provide health care services to individual patients and the surrounding community as a whole. All three obligations are important, but the creation of new doctors is the core function of a med school and it is here that our current institutions are lacking.

To be of real value to society, physicians need to have knowledge, skills, training and empathy. However, it is empathy that distinguishes a profession from a trade – and that quality should be part of what is required to obtain a med school diploma. In other words, med schools exist to fulfill societal needs, not the individual desires of professors and administrators and the students who learn to be doctors there. Like our other health care institutions, med schools have been corrupted by money and they are transmitting that disease. This needs to stop.

We are going to build a number of new medical schools in the coming years. Our population is growing, and aging, and we need all the things that med schools can provide. But we also need our med schools to conceptualize health care differently, to re-examine and renew their value systems, and to graduate physicians who regard their profession as a calling that involves personal sacrifice for the greater good. I don't know if the entrenched inhabitants of our current med schools are willing to change, but I believe we have an opportunity to insist that new med schools behave differently. We – all of us – can exert our influence by getting involved and making our voices heard. In order to be built, med schools have to obtain a variety of permits. Just as environmental groups inject themselves into the permitting process on various projects, so should we when it comes to new med schools. Med schools take public money in a variety of forms, which means that if there's a new school planned for your state or community, you have the opportunity to request that your elected officials push for explicit assurances that ethics and empathy be part of the school's overall mission statement and academic curriculum. Med schools mount fund-raising campaign, which means that you have the opportunity to ask donors to make their contributions contingent on the school placing mission before margin. Doing these things can put positive pressure on the entire system. As always, real change won't be easy or swift. But if we don't change the value systems of physicians at their source, where do we change them?

Chapter Nine

WHY WE HAVE TO RATION HEALTHCARE AND HOW TO DO IT COMPASSIONATELY

If We Spend Our Health Care Dollars More Wisely, We Can Meet Everyone's Needs

Many years ago, as a primary care physician at small Idaho hospital, I delivered twin boys who were two months premature and in critical condition. As they were taken to the neonatal ward, I conferred with the pediatrician and other members of the medical team assembled for the birth. Our conclusion was quick and unanimous: the babies had to be transferred immediately to a larger, better equipped hospital in Salt Lake City. We told the parents what they had to do and they agreed.

One infant died a couple days later. The other one, although he survived, was rendered blind and retarded, among other issues, by the extensive treatment required to keep him alive. His long and enormously expensive hospitalization, with the mother moving to Salt Lake City to be near her baby, ruined the family financially. They wound up in bankruptcy court, the mother nearly suicidal, the marriage strained almost to the point of breaking.

Because their organs and systems are not fully developed, preemies are highly vulnerable, and the life-sustaining treatment they receive quite often results in them being severely handicapped. I knew that, as did the other members of the medical team.

I had been a doctor for about 10 years at that point and was well acquainted with the parents. I had delivered their two previous children without incident and they trusted me. But in this situation I never gave them the opportunity to make a different choice. They could have chosen to let us treat their babies right there. We were not without resources, and that would have kept the family united to face whatever happened together. Instead, physicians decided that these babies needed the ultimate in medical care, even though that care was almost 200 miles away.

Like other members of the medical establishment, I was trained – indoctrinated really – to do everything medically possible to keep those infants alive. We swung into action, steamrolling the dazed parents, without any real reflection on what the collateral consequences of our decision might be, or what alternatives were available.

This tragedy, which remains in my consciousness more than 30 years later, was one of the events that prompted me to begin thinking about the assumptions and motivations driving the way we deliver health care in this country. Like most doctors, then and now, I had proceeded essentially on the autopilot mentality of doing what was indicated scientifically without any regard for the ripple effects our decisions had on the patients and their families. It was almost as if they were experiments in a Petri dish.

Looking back, I believe that I could have and should have provided the parents with more information and helped them with the very difficult choices they faced. There were no "right" answers, but the parents didn't know anything about the probabilities, consequences and costs of the choices open to them. Perhaps they would have made the same decisions, perhaps not, but they never really had the chance. We rushed them down a road that ultimately led to their financial ruin.

America is on that same road today. Healthcare is accounting for an ever-increasing percentage of our GDP and as we know – both from personal experience and credible surveys – we're not spending that money wisely or well. Like those parents, we are not making healthcare decisions – either individually or as a society – with our eyes open and with consideration for all of the consequences. As a result, we have the worst of both worlds – the overall quality of American healthcare is declining at the same time its cost is rising sharply. Left unchecked, healthcare spending will eventually crowd out other vital social and ethical priorities. The current trajectory of healthcare spending is simply not sustainable. We've got to manage our healthcare costs more intelligently, and there's no way to do that without confronting the stark reality of rationing.

Before delving further into this highly charged issue, I want to be clear about something. We have to ration healthcare because it is the right thing to do, the ethical thing to do, not because it will save money, although that does matter. If we ration healthcare ethically and compassionately, in an informed manner that considers both the needs of the individual and of society as a whole, and it winds up being 20% of GDP, then so be it. I believe, however, that costs would decline. In fact, I believe allocating healthcare rationally, which is another way to think about rationing, would save us enough to provide basic coverage to most and possibly even all of the approximately 46 million people in this country who do not have health insurance.

Healthcare obviously cannot be 100% of GDP, or anywhere close. The same is true for education, defense, or other high-priority items. Healthcare is a finite resource, and we need to ration it ethically because misallocation of a limited resource that people must have to survive is cruel and immoral. Allocating healthcare the way we currently do, based largely on who's got the most money and who's going to make the most money, is pretty close to criminal.

We misallocate healthcare because of a number of factors, but a major reason is our unquestioning emphasis on doing everything medically that can possibly be done – regardless of whether that's what the patient really wants. This blind allegiance to science at the expense of compassion is particularly true at the beginning and end of life, periods where we spend enormous amounts of money on treatments of dubious value. Because people at these stages are helpless themselves (and often beyond our ability to help) our hearts go out to them. Quite often, we respond by subjecting them to futile care that includes extremely unpleasant and expensive procedures – without stopping to think about whether what we are doing is really in their best interests. Part of it, I believe, is that we assuage our own feelings of helplessness, loss and grief by taking action. This is certainly true of many families who demand that physicians "do something" for their terminally ill parent – and it is often true for the physicians as well.

Premature babies cannot tell us what they want, of course, but I have often wondered what they would say if they could. If they could comprehend the statistics, which quite clearly show that treatments given to the prematurely born result in a much higher incidence of retardation and severely disabling diseases, would they choose to be treated? We cannot know, so we act, and the collateral consequences are often horrendous, as in the example I have given. I could give many others.

We often do know – and trample on – the wishes of those at the other end of life, the terminally ill and severely impaired patients whose over-riding wish is to die with as much peace and dignity as they can. The hospital environment, with its often-frantic pace and built-in bias for action, does not lend itself to candid, thoughtful discussions about whether it's time to stop treatment and let nature take its course. Moreover, our system pays doctors to do procedures, not to counsel patients and their families about the realities of dying, and once the patient starts down the road of aggressive intervention it's very difficult to halt that process. The reality is that many aggressive treatments are, from the patient's point of view, often worse than the disease and wind up prolonging what is by then a miserable existence.

Because we're not in their situation ourselves, it can be difficult to understand and accept when an elderly loved one tells us that he or she doesn't want any more treatment. And although many elderly patients cling desperately to life, others have re-organized the way they think about life. If you realize that you're never going to be able to live independently again, that what lies ahead is an unknown length of time in a disabled and often painful state, life looks very different. These patients understand, as their families and physicians often do not, that allowing death to occur is not the same as causing death to occur, and they want to be able to go. This is the time when hospice care, which can be provided wherever the patient is living, can be so valuable in helping all the parties accept the inevitable and go there with as much dignity and comfort as possible.

Again, I speak from experience. In the later years of his life, my father suffered from chronic obstructive pulmonary disease (COPD). After a lifetime of vitality, all he could do was watch TV, go for a drive and sometimes a short walk, his oxygen bottle always present. He knew he wasn't going to get better and he knew full well that the end was near. He had accepted both those realities when, as is often the case with COPD, a minor respiratory illness sent him into the ICU with pulmonary failure.

Patients in the condition my father had reached can be kept alive in the hospital for quite a while with a device that fits over their face and forces oxygen into their lungs. However, the device is very uncomfortable and hard to bear. In addition, when COPD patients get to that point, it's very rare for them to ever leave the hospital. Nonetheless, the attending doctors and staff kept forcing the device and accompanying treatment onto my father, which eventually led him to plead with me.

"I didn't realize it was this hard to die," he said. "Please keep that stuff away from me."

I made sure that his wishes were followed, sat with him and watched him die. It wasn't easy for either of us, but it was what he wanted, and what was just.

The medical profession was very kind and helpful to my father during his life and as his disability progressed. However, it's the capacity to meet a patient's needs in times of stress, under difficult conditions, that shows whether or not physicians are really good at their profession. Here is where the medical profession failed my father, as I believe I failed the family with the premature twins. Physicians have also failed our society as a whole, by allowing a disease-oriented focus to prevail over a patient-oriented focus, by thinking more about what we are getting paid than whether what we are doing is really the best thing for the patient, and by letting slick malpractice lawyers and a corrupt political and legal system exert far too much influence on medical decision-making.

As I noted in an earlier chapter, this failure extends to medical schools, which by and large emphasize scientific aptitude and procedural skills over human qualities like compassion and integrity. One result of this orientation is that enormous amounts of money are spent by academic research centers on elderly patients in the end stages of life. These centers, which offer the most advanced procedures and most renowned specialists, tend to attract patients and families who want everything that possibly can be done to be done. The accompanying tabs are huge and Medicare, which ultimately means you and I, often pays the bill. That may be all right with you, but do you recall anyone asking?

I have chosen these two examples because I was there to witness what happened, because together they represent an inordinate amount of healthcare spending – and also because they are laden with the emotions that any discussion of healthcare rationing inevitably arouses. There are thousand upon thousands of other similar instances, less dramatic perhaps but nonetheless significant in the aggregate, where we misuse our healthcare dollars.

Health care cannot provide everything to everyone – we simply don't have the resources. Moreover, when we spend some of our limited dollars on futile care and treatments of questionable value, we cannot spend those dollars in areas that have an enormous payoff – preventive care is a prime example. If we redirected a fraction of what we spend on futile care into preventive care, the payoff in terms of relieving human pain and suffering would be enormous. And while terms like "cost-effectiveness" and "payoff" may sound cold and impersonal when we're talking about someone lying in a hospital bed, there are tradeoffs in healthcare just as there are in other areas of life.

When you step back and look at it in the context of the greatest good for the greatest number, the logic of rationing health care is irrefutable. But, as always, the devil is in the details, and as soon as it's our loved one who's not going to get the wonder drug or surgical intervention, logic goes out the window and we're back in the jungle. This is why any discussion of rationing has to occur well away from the heat of the moment. The decisions we make on this issue – both individually and as a society – should be well-considered, not made in haste and under the duress of pain, fear and the pressure of health care providers who may have other agendas. That's not happening, so let's look at why.

Having a serious discussion about rationing health care is difficult for many reasons, but I believe one of the biggest is that it forces us to confront our own mortality. No matter how many amazing surgeries and miracle drugs are developed, I'm going to die. You too. Learning to live with the reality that our life will end is a major step toward true maturity and one that many people never take. Rationing brings us right up against that reality, so it's easy to understand why we don't want to talk about it. Mortality generally enters our conversations in times of crisis, often when a loved one is close to death or some event has rubbed our own noses in the fact that our days are numbered. Unfortunately, our country is in a health care crisis right now. It may not clutch at our hearts the same way a near-fatal accident or the death of a sibling does, but it's very real. If it were a hospital patient, our healthcare system would be in the ICU and the prognosis would be grim.

There are other reasons why we avoid the rationing discussion. For one thing, our politicians know that to suggest systematically denying health care to anyone, which is how their opponents would immediately frame it, is to commit electoral suicide. Many of them understand quite well that we have to ration health care, but they view saying so as the equivalent of going out on a limb and then sawing it off. We're not going to get any leadership on this issue from Washington. The lies, half-truths and manipulations deployed by our politicians on health care issues as they struggle to win office are cynical and shameful.

The same holds true for other sectors where thoughtful and well-informed people could bring this issue to the fore. As I have mentioned, the medical-industrial complex now accounts for about one-sixth of our economy and many millions of jobs. Although some academic health care theorists have broached the subject, we're not going to hear much about rationing from within the medical-industrial complex for the simple reason that limiting or reducing the amount we spend on health care translates into fewer jobs and less money for those who feed on the current system.

Because our health care delivery system is so distorted, with individual financial responsibility displaced onto employers and government, the enormous amounts of money we spend on futile care doesn't seem like a pressing issue. It is. For example, about 60% of all Medicare expenditures go for patients in their last six weeks of life. Is that what we want as a society? Is that a conscious, well-informed, vigorously debated choice we've made? Remember, every dollar spent on keeping someone alive for an extra week is a dollar that can't be spent on vaccinating your grandchildren, replacing your hip, or (you fill in the blank). When California taxpayers spent some $1 million on a heart transplant for a 31-year-old prison inmate – a twice-convicted felon who was serving a 14-year sentence for armed robbery – that was $1 million that couldn't be spent on (fill in that blank too). This matters to everyone. It's the reality of how our limited resources are being allocated today in our health care system, and we've got to talk about it.

Although other countries do ration health care, with varying degrees of patient satisfaction, the only large scale attempt to do so within the U.S. occurred in Oregon, which in 1994 began rationing health care for its Medicaid population. The intent of the program was to expand Medicaid to cover all Oregon residents below the poverty level, paying for the increase by denying coverage for certain medical services deemed less valuable than others.

Oregon looked to its citizens (what a concept) for input in determining which services were more or less valuable than others, holding a series of town meetings at which the topic was discussed. In general, the citizens felt that basic health care for all should take precedence over heroic measures for the few. In prioritizing health care services above the basic level, some of the determining values that emerged were prevention, cost-effectiveness, quality of life, length of life, and functionality. Ultimately, the state produced a "priority list" of 709 medical treatments and said its Medicaid program would no longer pay for those ranked below No. 587. Among other benefits, this cutoff helped Oregon to provide basic health care services to an additional 100,000 residents, reduce the percentage of its uninsured population, reduce uncompensated care in hospitals and reduce the use of hospital emergency rooms for routine care.

The Oregon rationing experiment produced howls of outrage (and lawsuits) from various rights groups and eventually was rejected by the U.S. Department of Health and Human Services (Medicaid is administered by the states but paid for by the Feds). HHS said that Oregon's rationing program discriminated against people with disabilities and cited a number of examples. One was that Oregon's list would have denied life support to extremely low birth weight babies under 23 weeks' gestation, a situation I have already discussed. Another was that the state refused to cover liver transplants for people with cirrhosis of the liver resulting from alcoholism. HHS viewed this as discriminatory on the grounds that alcoholism was "a disabling condition." Again, bear in mind that what this essentially means is that you and I as taxpayers are supposed to pay for liver transplants for alcoholics. Does that make sense to you? Do you remember voting on that?

Oregon's program did not survive, but it did leave behind lessons for us, lessons that are even more pertinent now than they were then. One is that medical treatments can be prioritized. We may argue over how and where the lines should be drawn, but they can be drawn. Another lesson is that the public (patients) must be involved in the decision-making process. Physicians and other qualified medical authorities should play a major role, of course, but when it comes to the values that ultimately will determine the priority of health care treatments, that's not solely the province of "experts." Just as the parents of the premature twins I mentioned at the beginning of this chapter should have been involved in the decisions regarding their children, so should parents all over the country be involved in deciding how our health care dollars should be spent. We all should be involved.

Another lesson is that no matter what decisions are made and where the lines are drawn, someone is going to be unhappy, either immediately or later on when their particular situation isn't covered. There's no way around this. If we accept the premise that we do not have unlimited resources for health care, we have to also accept that not everyone is going to get everything they want. Maybe that means the convict doesn't get a heart transplant and the alcoholic doesn't get a new liver. Maybe the choices are not quite so clear-cut and the decisions are difficult and heart-rending. And maybe it's you or me who doesn't get what we want. That's what we're talking about here – some individuals don't get everything they want in order that we may provide health care services that generate the greatest good for the greatest number.

We also need to acknowledge that even with a carefully and compassionately designed rationing program, there will still be those who can purchase whatever health care services they want simply because they have the money to do so. There's no way around this either. Life isn't fair and we cannot make it so. However, we can reform our healthcare system in ways that place a higher value on care that benefits the many rather than the few, that use this finite resource more wisely, and that recognize and honor the wishes and dignity of the individual.

Prioritizing – and then rationing – health care according to a set of values similar to those developed in Oregon will not be a short or simple process. It will require that we think of others and place their interests on essentially the same level as our own. It will require real change on the part of physicians and medical schools.

It will face opposition from a variety of entrenched interest groups who are doing quite well under the current system. It will mean making difficult choices and living with those choices when they become personal rather than abstract. And it will mean thinking and acting in advance instead of hoping that somehow we won't have to make difficult decisions.

As is usually the case, the process should begin with the individual. Having a relationship with a primary care physician within the context of a medical home can facilitate the process of thinking about these weighty topics and making informed decisions. For example, if you have not created an advanced directive that tells your doctor what kind of medical treatment you want if you are unable to make decisions on your own, I urge you to discuss this with your doctor and put your wishes down in writing. This can spare you and your loved ones from heightening and prolonging the pain that often accompanies the end of life. If you want every possible treatment and life-sustaining intervention, by all means say so. The point is to consider these issues ahead of time and try to plan as best you can. The same holds true for parents and their minor children, and adult children and their parents. Don't put these matters off – talk to those concerned about what you want, what they want, and how you might fulfill those wishes. If your doctor won't spend time talking to you about these issues, get another doctor. You have the right – and the responsibility – to make thoughtful, unhurried, informed decisions about the medical treatment you receive.

Once you have worked through these issues on a personal level, you will have a foundation for discussing how health care should be allocated (rationed) on a larger scale – within your family, community, state and nation. You may need to take the lead initiating those discussions, because leaving these matters to politicians, lobbyists, insurance companies, academic "experts" and physician groups is what's left us where we are today.

Ultimately, this is a question of values, not techniques and procedures and premiums and co-pays. Our health care system is in ruins primarily because it was built on the wrong values – greed, selfishness, denial and dishonesty are just some that come to mind. We – meaning you and I and the folks across the street – are going to have to rebuild it on a new set of values. Those values must reflect the needs of the individual patient and of society as a whole – all within the framework of the reality that health care is a finite resource and must therefore be rationed. The sooner we get started on that discussion, the closer we will be to creating a new health care system that works.

Chapter Ten

RE-IMAGINING HEALTH CARE

*How to Re-conceptualize the System We've Already Got
So That Patients, Providers and Payers Can All Benefit*

If you have stayed with me this far, I hope you will by now agree that what we have today in American health care is not a "system" but a contradictory contraption of wired-together parts that don't mesh, pull in opposing directions and are pretty close to coming apart. The question, of course, is what should we do about it, and it is here that we splinter into dozens of groups, each coalesced largely around self-interest and ideology rather than acknowledging the overriding principle that health care exists for patients. These groups have been battling each other for years, enriching lawyers, lobbyists, "do-gooder" foundations, ad agencies, PR firms, media outlets and various others. Meanwhile, American health care has declined in quality, increased in cost, and become more dysfunctional and impersonal. Not only is our "system" not working – our efforts to fix it aren't working either!

As we have seen, what we have was never thought through or designed – it bumped and lurched along, impacted by historical accidents such as job-based health insurance, well-meant but ill-executed governmental programs such as Medicare and Medicaid, the rise of a vast medical-industrial complex whose members initially served patients but morphed into profit-driven machines, "market-driven" movements such as managed care, myriad scientific advances, and various other factors. Paralleling and interacting with these elements was what I view as a widespread erosion of our societal values, an ethical and moral decline that has brought us to a place where our gods are greed, power, and unbridled self-interest. We – the patients – have become bystanders, afterthoughts, accidental ingredients.

It is the confluence of these things that give rise to the obscene spectacles of health care industry CEOs taking home millions of dollars while patients who desperately need medical care go without it or go bankrupt paying for it. What kind of society are we when pensioners are cutting their pills in halves and quarters to stretch their prescriptions while the CEOs of the drug companies making those medications are paid $1 million a week and more? In re-imagining health care, we need also to re-examine our moral values.

In addressing the question of what kind of health care system we want, let's begin with an area of common ground. We may each differ in many ways – income, the current state of our health, insurance coverage, political ideology are just some – but we all share one important characteristic: we are all patients. Therefore, in re-imagining health care, in trying to conceptualize what our system would look like if it actually made sense, let's start with these kinds of questions: What really matters to patients? What's the best way to provide patients with what really matters to them? How do we deliver quality care to patients while being open about the reality that not everyone can have everything they want? And most important, what should be the foundational values of our health care system?

I have the honor to be chairing a task force for the Accreditation Association for Ambulatory Health Care on what is now being called the Medical Home, which I believe is the wave of the future in health care. Ironically, it is also in many respects how medicine was practiced 50 years ago, when patients were truly the focus and primary care physicians were the dominant practitioners. If we could, and I think we can, combine the values of those days with the enormous advances medicine has made since then, we would have an excellent health care system. Isn't that worth pursuing, and vigorously?

As the name implies, the Medical Home takes the focus of health care away from greed and profits, which is where it currently all too often lies, and places that focus on patients – the common ground I just referenced. From the point of view of the patient, here are what I see as the core elements and principles of the Medical Home:

- Every patient should have an open and ongoing relationship with a primary care physician of their choice who is their first point of contact, sees them regularly and coordinates all of their care, delegating as appropriate to specialists, staff members within the practice and other professionals who can respond to the patient's needs.
- Every patient should be able to choose their own personal physician based not on whether the physician is on an insurance company or HMO roster, but solely on the factors that matter to the patient – factors such as trust, empathy, and availability.

- Every patient should be treated according to a whole-person orientation that includes care across all stages of life and encompasses preventive services as well as acute, chronic and end-of-life care. This orientation should promote "wellness" in a pro-active manner.
- Every patient should have access to their primary care physician and to health care that also includes other communications channels such as email, phone consultations and websites that offer information useful to the individual patient. What those channels are and how and when they are used should be discussed and agreed upon by each patient and physician.
- Every patient should have an Electronic Medical Record (EMR) that is secure, current, comprehensive and available to providers and payers, as the patient chooses. This EMR should be portable, so that patients can download it and take their records wherever they wish.
- Every patient should be covered by portable health insurance that compensates the Medical Home according to a monthly per-patient fee schedule (capitation) that recognizes the value of whole-person, longitudinal health care, as well as the benefits of continuity and health care delivered by all members of the team led by the patient's primary care physician.

Making this "wish list" into reality obviously is going to require tectonic changes in the way health care is currently conceptualized, delivered and financed, and I have no illusions about how difficult that will be. However, our task in this chapter is to "re-imagine health care" as it should be. We must be pragmatic, but at the same time, if we don't know where we want to go, we have no hope of getting there. Moreover, if you accept my premise that meaningful health care reform is not going to come from a corrupt and co-opted Washington, nor from well-heeled and well-fed members of the investor-owned, for-profit medical-industrial complex, then where is it going to come from?

The only answer, I submit, is that health care reform must originate with patients. If you step back far enough and look at the situation realistically, it cannot be otherwise. Every other group in the health care picture, and I sadly must acknowledge that this includes too many doctors, has an axe to grind, turf to protect, and profits to preserve. When we turn to the powers that be, we're asking the foxes to come up with a better way of managing the henhouse. But once we as patients really get that, once we realize that no one is going to solve the health care mess except us, then that truth can set us free and generate enormous power. Collectively, we are far stronger than the entrenched forces that seek to protect the status quo, but we must understand and agree as a group on what health care should look like before we can unite to change things.

I will have more to say about how patients can become a positive societal force for health care reform in the next chapter, but I want first to expand on the above principles and explain why they are so critically important. In so doing, I hope to build consensus and support for these principles that can translate into an agenda for positive change.

A fundamental reality of health care, and one we have lost sight of, is that quality medicine is practiced one-on-one. A competent primary care physician who has developed a trusting relationship with a patient can quickly determine when something is amiss and move expeditiously to respond. The evidence is right there, in the form of the patient's medical record, the personal knowledge the physician has gained about the patient during the trusting relationship that exists between them, and, most importantly, in the human interaction between two people who are trying to answer the question: "What's wrong?" There are all kinds of expensive studies demonstrating that you get better health care outcomes and lower costs when doctor and patient have an ongoing relationship, but it's really just common sense.

One of the biggest benefits to patients from an ongoing relationship is that it can save us from the dreary merry-go-round of tests and specialists that is so easily set in motion under the current system. The examining room where patient and doctor meet is also a fork in the road. Down one path lies perfectly good but minimally invasive (and less costly) care. Down the other lies an open-ended process that all too often is unpleasant, expensive and unproductive. A primary care physician who knows you can spare you some of that because medicine is ultimately about probabilities. People generally don't like to hear it put this way (and doctors won't say it this way), but if I know you, I can make a much, much better guess as to what might be ailing you. If I'm seeing you for the first time, I'm going to want the confirmation and comfort of tests and specialists.

Another reality of medicine is that perhaps half of all patients who enter the examining room with a complaint are not physically sick. They're afraid they're going to get sick. Basically, it's stress. The best medicine they can receive is a little time spent with a physician who knows them, listens to them, demonstrates that he/she cares about them, and helps them cope with what is really wrong. But the same dynamics apply – if

I know you, I can supply what you need and help you stay on the right path.

An ongoing relationship also supplies the foundation to deal with yet another reality of medicine, which is that most diseases that kill people are rooted in the personal lifestyle choices they make. Smoking, excessive drinking, obesity and other forms of self-destructive behavior can be addressed by a patient's trusted personal physician in a way that a one-time encounter simply cannot. As a doctor from the "old school," I take this train of thought even further, believing that a primary care physician should monitor, encourage and support patients and families in their need to have appropriate physical activity, nutrition, self-care/emotional health, sleep, spirituality, personal relationships, and even positive financial habits. That may seem intrusive to some, but after treating thousands of patients I can assure you that these things are inter-related and bear directly on a person's overall health.

Just as there are many situations that can best be handled directly and immediately by the patient's primary care physician, there are also many situations which can't. In such cases, a specialist should be called in for a consult, which is basically an informed opinion; or the patient should be referred to a specialist for care of the specific issue. However, the care provided by the specialist should be coordinated by the patient's personal physician in the Medical Home. By definition, not to mention training and mindset, specialists are not whole-person oriented. They are disease and procedure-oriented. But everything a physician does for a patient has consequences that go beyond the immediate treatment objective, and this is where so many people get into trouble today. Contra-indicated medications are perhaps the most familiar issue here, but they are just part of the story. When you start treating a patient, especially for anything serious, you inevitably disrupt their body's systems. The initial decision to treat must take this into account, but the consequences – and they are often multifaceted and ongoing – must be monitored and responded to as indicated. Again, this is something best overseen by the patient's primary care physician, who has a fuller picture of the patient's overall health and who will be seeing the patient long after the specialist has moved on.

The same principle – coordination of a patient's care should be handled by that patient's primary care physician – holds true for other types of providers, both individual and institutional. During the course of their relationship, a patient will receive health care services from many sources besides their primary care physician. A partial list might encompass lab and hospital staffers, home health care providers, medical technicians, physical therapists, patient support groups, and so on. This is as it should be – there are many levels of health care. The role of the primary care physician, in addition to treating the patient directly, should be to act as the leader of a team that provides different types and levels of care based on the needs of each patient. If those resources are available within the physician's practice, they can be delivered directly; if they are not, the physician can assemble them and oversee their delivery.

Experience has shown me repeatedly how quickly things can go wrong when care is not delivered through this model. I recall an instance involving a young woman who was working hard at her college studies when she fell in love with a young man. The couple moved in together. The stresses and adjustments of the new relationship, added to the stress of school, began to affect the woman. She sought help from a psychiatrist who, after seeing her only briefly, told her she was too reliant and dependent on her family. The solution? Distance yourself from your family. The woman did as she was counseled and the results were swift. She wound up in the hospital. This brought her primary care physician into the picture – for the first time. Her physician, who knew her, knew her family, knew the psychiatrist, and knew the family relationship was not the issue, changed the marching orders immediately. He got her away from the psychiatrist and under the care of a different psychiatrist. It's now many years later and the woman has done quite well in her personal and professional life. But it almost went very bad indeed, and the reason was simple. Someone who didn't know the situation put the patient on the wrong course – and this has almost certainly happened again during the time it took you to read this paragraph.

Although the reasons I have just advanced for everyone having a personal physician deal primarily with the benefits to the patient, there are also very significant societal advantages to this approach. Multiplied by many thousands of doctors and millions of patients, the fork in the road I described earlier –effective but minimally invasive treatment or the specialist/test/procedure merry-go-round – has enormous implications for our nation's overall health costs. The same is true for preventive/wellness health care – if a substantial number of patients could be steered towards healthier lifestyles, the savings would be profound, both in human and financial terms. But as things stand now, many insurers really don't want to pay for preventive care because the payoff in terms of lower expenses for chronic illness often comes years down the line and they're afraid that by then some other insurer (or Medicare) will reap the benefit. That's just one consequence of a value system based on profits rather than patients.

I can't prove it, but I truly believe that we could halt the increase in health care costs simply by making this first element of the Medical Home (having a primary care physician that the patient trusts) the rule rather than the exception. The patients I cared for missed less work, made quicker recoveries, got the care they needed earlier, and understood more about their health issues and how to respond to them. That wasn't because I was a miracle worker; it was because I had ongoing relationships with them and could help them get well and stay well.

The second element, making it possible for every patient to be able to choose their personal physician based on the factors that matter to them, also has significant benefits to both the individual patient and society as a whole. Patient satisfaction with an individual physician is based on a number of factors, including the perceived competence of the physician, whether the physician is sensitive to the patient's culture and ethnicity, how accessible the physician is, how the front office behaves and the patient's trust in them as professionals. But the overwhelming factor, across all cultures, age groups, income levels and types of disease, is whether the patient feels that the physician cares about them as a person, which is essentially the definition of empathy.

After many thousands of encounters with many thousands of patients, I can tell you that there's a chemistry/spark/bond – call it what you will – that sometimes is there between doctor and patient and sometimes is not. If it is, amazing things can happen. If it's not, neither party is likely to be very satisfied. But the real point here is that the patient should be able to make a free choice in the matter. If health care really were the free market many ideologues contend it is (or should be), that's what would happen. It's what should happen. Let patients vote with their feet, as the saying goes.

When there's a human connection between doctor and patient, all sorts of other things happen to how health care is provided. Patients open up more, so the physician has a better chance of discovering something earlier. Patients are more compliant – meaning they take their meds as prescribed or follow whatever other treatment regimen the physician has recommended – and guess what? The patient does better, which in medicalese means you get better outcomes. Again, you multiply this by enough doctors and enough patients and you get a significant improvement in overall outcomes, meaning that as a society we have greater success in addressing our health care problems.

The third element of the Medical Home is treating every patient according to a whole-person orientation that includes care across all stages of life and encompasses preventive services as well as acute, chronic and end-of-life care. A whole-person orientation, as I mentioned above, recognizes that treating a patient inevitably involves making judgments about benefit and risk. Rather than focusing just on a specific issue, a good primary care physician will look at that issue in the context of the whole person. Every medication, indeed every treatment, has consequences, side effects. If I treat a depressed or hypertensive patient "successfully" according to certain benchmarks but in the process damp down their mental faculties to the point where they are sleepwalking through their lives, is that good care? Obviously the answer is no, but don't think for a moment that I'm stacking the deck – there are countless examples of patients having one issue "solved" to the detriment of their overall quality of life. Believe me, these kinds of questions are not asked as often as they should be. Payers, including Medicare,

Medicaid and the dominant HMO accrediting organization, the National Committee on Quality Assurance, think primarily in terms of percentages and what works for a given "population" and not nearly enough about individual patients. Quality health care is delivered one-on-one, not by relying on batting averages.

A whole-person, longitudinal (regularly over a long time period) approach also offers a much better opportunity to combat chronic illness, because the origins of many chronic diseases are rooted in patient lifestyles. A physician whose caring behavior over a period of some years has engendered trust and respect in his/her patient can have a far more significant impact on the patient's behavior than someone the patient is only going to see once or twice. We don't need any studies to tell us this; it's another example of common sense. But again, multiply this individual relationship-based opportunity by millions of patients and you get an enormous impact. The American Public Health Association estimates that chronic illness (heart disease, diabetes, obesity) accounts for about 75% of all health care costs. Modify the behavior of just 20% of the population and the savings run into the billions.

Our society – and consequently our health care system – glorifies youth, devalues aging and makes a good show of denying the ultimate reality that we're all going to die. But these stages of life are inescapable and should be an integral part of how health care is provided. Helping patients deal with the infirmities of age and the inevitability of death can be acts of great kindness, but this is difficult if not impossible with episodic health care, which is what we have now.

The fourth element involves providing patients with enhanced access to health care, which includes being able to see your doctor readily but also takes into account the fact that you don't always need to. There are plenty of occasions when other communications channels such as email, phone consultations and self-management information via a website will do just fine. Here again, it is the perception and desires of the patient that should determine what "enhanced access" means. Patients shouldn't have to put up with a physician and/or medical group that's open 8:30 to 5:30 and shunts them off to the ER or Urgent Care at any other time. They should be able to vote with their feet and find a Medical Home, something our current health insurance system doesn't allow.

I should note in passing that, over time, enhanced access does reduce overall costs. My time spent treating patients has persuaded me that the anxiety surrounding either illness or the fear of illness is exacerbated when the patient does not have an established, comfortable relationship with a physician. Years ago, I shared call coverage with two other doctors. One of the physician's practice style was the antithesis of a Medical Home. He was a "catch me if you can" doctor – available for urgent issues but not generally accessible to his patients. That was just his nature. Both I and my other partner were easily accessible – it was a value we believed in deeply. But what happened was the opposite of what you might expect. The two of us got fewer after-hours calls than our partner who was less accessible. Our patients knew they could get to us if they really needed to, and somehow that meant they didn't really need to nearly as often. The patient demographics and other features of the practice were the same, so the difference, I believe, was the comfort level of our patients. Simply put, they felt better because they knew we were available. The same dynamic holds true today for my physician children. Their patients know they can get to them, and because of that the patients rarely call after hours (when they do, it's usually a call that should have been made – and their patients get a prompt response).

In addressing the subject of Electronic Medical Records (EMRs), the fifth element, let me begin with a few statistics. According to a 1999 Institute of Medicine study, as many as 98,000 American die each year as a result of preventable medical errors, meaning that the U.S. health care system itself is perhaps the fifth-leading cause of the death in our country. Another 1.5 million patients are harmed every year by errors in medications. Almost a third of the more than 3 billion prescriptions written each year by doctors require a follow-up with the dispensing pharmacy for clarification. More than 90% of those prescriptions are transmitted using a 5,000-year-old technology: pen and paper.

I could continue, but the point should be obvious. We've got to standardize and digitize patient medical records in a way that lets patients understand their own health information and gives them control over who they share it with. This would reduce errors, cut costs and improve the overall quality of health care by ensuring that everyone is working from the same page. Computerized systems can flag incorrect dosages, note when a new medication might cause conflicts with a patent's existing prescriptions, aid in diagnosing, provide physicians with quick access to the latest research on a specific condition ... the list goes on and on.

The specter of Big Brother (or insurance companies) illegally accessing and misusing patients' medical information is real and must be confronted, but the benefits of EMRs are far too great to let this stop us. The technology to collect, store and make comprehensive and current EMRs available to patients, providers and payers already exists – we just have to use it.

Many organizations already are – the Veterans Administration has a unified and fully integrated system that give its physicians instant access to the records of more than 5.5 million patients. Many large health care organizations also have sophisticated health information technology (HIT) systems.

One reason that we haven't moved faster on this front is that physicians aren't compensated for converting those bulky paper files to digital form. A basic EMR system can easily cost a small group practice $50,000 to $100,000, and that comes right out of the physicians' hide. In an age where physicians who are trying to move to the Medical Home model are woefully undercompensated, EMRs are simply not feasible financially. There is also resistance, primarily among older physicians, to learning how to use computerized systems, although this is rapidly disappearing. Another obstacle is that we haven't achieved what the tech folks call "interoperability" – meaning that the different EMR systems being used by the physician, the lab, the imaging center and all the other players can talk to each other. One of the big reasons we haven't achieved interoperability is that rather than cooperating, the major EMR companies are busily fighting with each other in an attempt to make their system dominant. They know this is going to be a huge "market" and they all envision themselves as the Microsoft of EMRs. Their focus is on profits and meanwhile, preventable errors are killing almost 100,000 patients every year. Is there something wrong with this picture?

What is perhaps the biggest obstacle to EMRs – patients' fears that they will lose control over their health care records – can and must be addressed. With plentiful news stories about credit records being stolen and top-secret laptop computers being left on the bus, you can certainly see why patients are concerned. But the technology to encrypt EMRs already exists, and does anyone really think paper records are somehow safer? We can mandate that payers not be allowed to use EMRs to deny coverage and deal with similar concerns. There are security and privacy issues, yes, but they can be worked through. When we do that, patients will embrace EMRs for the simple reason that they may just save their lives, not to mention their money.

This is another reform that would pay for itself as far as the system as a whole is concerned, so we must find a way to pass the savings on to physicians and others who have to make the initial investment in costly systems. A 2005 RAND study estimated that 90% adoption of EMRs nationwide would produce annual cost savings of about $77 billion; other studies have put the figure much higher. Pick your own number – the point is that EMRs save lives, improve health care and reduce costs.

The final element, health insurance, is a complex and contentious topic that has filled many a book by itself. But if we're going to reap the many benefits of the preceding elements – and among those benefits is a significant reduction in overall health care costs – we're going to have to find a way to compensate the Medical Home fairly for making those elements an everyday reality for patients. You can't just mandate that physicians adopt these practices without transforming the way in which they are reimbursed. That means our nation's health insurance system has to change in at least the following ways:

- Health insurance must be portable so that individuals take it with them when they change jobs, locations or physicians. Ultimately, that means it can't be employer-provided, as it is for most people now.

- The health insurance industry must become essentially a utility, allowed to earn a decent rate of return but required to pay a certain percentage of premium dollars back out to the patients/policyholders who are paying those premiums.
- The value of whole-person, coordinated, continuous health care, including preventive care, must be recognized financially by payers. Primary care physicians who provide this care must be compensated at levels which encourage medical students to choose primary care as their profession.
- Individuals must bear some of their health care costs directly. Our old friend moral hazard has to be acknowledged. There must be a connection between the amount of health care resources a person uses and what it costs that person. There also must be a financial connection, a penalty if you will, between behaviors that necessitate the use of health care resources and what that use costs the patient. In other words, if you smoke, you should pay more for health insurance, because insurance and individual responsibility are inextricably linked. The flip side of insurance company greed is moral hazard. When people believe that someone else is paying for their health care, they want everything – cost and efficacy be damned. No pun intended, but consumers of health care have to have some skin in the game. Obviously, some people are better able to pay part of their way than others, and that issue has to be addressed. However, individual financial responsibility is a foundation on which we can promote the Medical Home, control expenses, use the most cost-effective therapies, and reign in excessive salaries and profits.

- The health insurance industry has to operate and be regulated on a national basis. One of the barriers to better health insurance is that the insurance industry is regulated not by one national authority but by each and every one of our 50 states (and the District of Columbia). As you can probably tell by now, I don't have a lot of sympathy for insurance companies, but making them jump through 51 sets of hoops doesn't make sense for anyone, including consumers. This antiquated regulatory system means, among other things, that a company might be required to cover a specific type of treatment in one state but not its neighbor. If you live in one state and work a few miles across the line in another, you could be covered for something by the health insurance you get on the job but be unable see a provider near your home because it's not covered there. Is there something wrong with this picture? State-by-state regulation also means that any type of innovative insurance product has to pass muster with 51 different regulators, each with its own approval process. The European Union, by contrast, is close to reaching agreement on establishing consistent regulations that would cover insurance companies in 27 different countries. We need a standardized set of regulations that will enable insurance carriers to provide health care insurance on a nationwide basis as Medicare does. Deciding on national standards for who and what should be covered and for how much is obviously going to be a gargantuan task, but again, what we have now just isn't working.

Most of all, we need to re-conceptualize what health insurance really is. I've mentioned repeatedly the three components of health care – patient, provider and payer. What's happened to us is that all these identities and roles have become subverted. Payers have become the providers, because it's the insurance companies and HMOs that decide which doctors you as a patient can see (through their rosters) and what treatment you as a patient can receive (through their approval processes). Providers, meanwhile, have become either hired hands, which is what most doctors are these days, or profit-driven entities (here I am referencing the members of the medical-industrial complex such as the publicly-held hospital chains or drug companies) whose primary motive is to drive profits as high as they can in the course of delivering health care.

Although most people don't completely realize it, largely because they get their health insurance on the job or from some government program, patients are really the payers. Whether it's directly in the form of checks you write, quasi-directly through the taxes you pay, or circuitously by way of individual compensation withheld by your employer for "company-paid" health insurance, it ultimately all comes back to you as the patient. Let's get rid of all the camouflage – one way or another, you and I are paying.

This is a central concept we have lost sight of when it comes to health insurance. Third-party payers have seized control of the health care system, making life-and-death decisions based not on medical knowledge nor on what's best for patients but on what's best for them! And who are they, really? It's our money, not theirs. The appropriate role of an insurance company is as a repository and recycler of premium dollars, nothing more. The core concept of insurance is that individuals in a given group need pay only a little to protect themselves if risk is spread among and borne by the group as a whole. There's no getting away from a certain level of administrative expenses, and there's nothing wrong with reasonable profits for the shareholders. However, the premiums we currently pay would be much lower if we removed the excessive and frequently outrageous costs of marketing, executive salaries, lavish overhead and other items.

We also need to move the decision-making on health care away from the insurers. Yes, decisions have to be made as to what is covered and what isn't, what is a "need" and what is a "want." But these are societal decisions, which should be informed by medical knowledge, weighed against the reality of finite health care resources, and made in the open forum of vigorous debate. Doctors and patients should be making these decisions collectively, not insurance company and HMO executives with one eye on their stock options.

I realize I'm treading on some cherished capitalist ideals here, and I have no illusions as to whether this kind of wrenching change will be easy or rapid. But in re-imagining health care, in moving towards a system that includes the elements I have set out, we have no choice but also to re-imagine how it's going to be paid for. As I discussed in the previous chapter, one of the things that means is rationing. Another is value judgments – collectively and fairly made, not mine or yours – on what constitutes a "need" and what defines a "want." Ultimately, I believe we have to provide everyone with what they truly need – a basic level of health care. To achieve this, everyone has to participate and everyone has to bear some of the costs. The exact formula – I would favor some kind of basic universal coverage combined with some form of Health Savings Accounts – is going to have to be thrashed out. If people who want additional health care services have the money to purchase them, they should be able to do so. Society doesn't have the obligation, not to mention the resources, to make life "fair."

Although much of what I've talked about in this chapter can be viewed as theoretical (hopefully leavened here and there with some doses of reality), it's really not an abstraction at all. Our health care system is a disgrace in no small part because we never sat down and thought about what it should look like. Instead, we just allowed it to evolve, or perhaps, devolve. This created a vacuum and what rushed to fill that vacuum were powerful forces that included the corporate profit motive, individual self-interest, professional lobbyists, government bumbling and bureaucracy, academic elitism, political ideology, tax policies, and various other factors. While we can't just blow up what has resulted, we also can't let it continue, for all the reasons I already have enumerated.

The model I have set out here isn't perfect, and I certainly encourage others to improve on it. My hope is that it can serve as a starting point for developing a grass-roots movement whereby patients take back control of the way they receive health care. By and large, patients respect their individual physicians (if they have one) but are outraged by the health care system as a whole. Without always being able to articulate it exactly, patients also understand that the root of the problem lies in the fact that payers are running the show. We need to reverse this. That means radical change, real reform. There's little point in applying another patch, which is essentially what most of the current proposals out there amount to. Instead, we as patients need to re-imagine health care. Because it's complex and intensely important, there's a tendency for us to defer to professional bodies and groups instead of thinking for ourselves. This is backwards, especially since many and perhaps most of these bodies are interested primarily in preserving and enlarging their own power and influence. In almost any other endeavor, the customer is king. That's how it should be in health care.

Chapter Eleven

WHAT EACH OF US CAN AND MUST DO TO RECLAIM CONTROL OF OUR HEALTH AND HEALTH CARE SYSTEM

Why Individual Ethics and Values Are the Answer to Our Health Care Problems

Coming to grips with – and acting upon – the realization that our own health and our nation's health care system are really individual responsibilities can be a difficult personal challenge. Everything seems so complicated, with all sorts of studies and government programs and mathematical formulas and academic experts who condescendingly convey the attitude that an ordinary person can't really grasp just how intricate individual health and our health care system really are.

Although there are legions of smart, well-connected and well-financed folks peddling this line, it simply isn't true. In terms of individual health, while genetics and luck play significant roles, most chronic diseases are rooted in lifestyle choices. As to our health care system, it is indeed complex, which enables all sorts of charlatans and scoundrels to hide out in its crevices while they rip us off. And because this complexity works to their financial advantage, many health care industry executives and other so-called experts denigrate the notion that reaching consensus on some fairly straightforward principles – and acting on them – would resolve most of the problems in our health care system. I'm not saying it's easy, but I am saying it's a lot simpler than we've been led to believe.

The reality is that we have much more power than we think we do. What we urgently have to do – all of us – is start exerting it. And while that's going to make some new demands on us, there's really no other choice. If you've stayed with me this long, and accept even half of what I've laid out, do you really believe that Washington politicians or the members of the medical-industrial complex are going to look out for you? As someone who's treated thousands of patients and toiled within the health care system for more than 40 years, trust me on this: you've got to take care of your own health and we've all got to take care of each other with regard to our health care system.

Let's start with what we each can do to take care of ourselves. As I mentioned, most of the diseases that damage quality of life and shorten life – diabetes, hypertension, strokes, heart disease, cancer, chronic obstructive pulmonary disease – spring from the specific choices you and I make every day. Here I'm talking about diet, exercise, sleep, emotional and financial stress, spirituality and all the other factors that in large part determine how we feel, whether we get sick, and how long we live. I'm well aware of all the societal forces that work against healthy lifestyle choices, but the fact that making good decisions isn't easy is not an argument for making bad ones. Smoking, alcohol and drug abuse, overeating, laziness and other behaviors can't be rationalized away. They also aren't "society's fault." Individual health is an individual responsibility.

There are hundreds of books and websites and other sources of material about healthy lifestyles, so I'm not going to get into specifics here other than to recommend common sense. For example, if you want to lose weight, eat less and move more. Don't fall for gimmick diets, which can really hurt you. Apply that same kind of simple, no-B.S., no excuses reasoning to your health habits and you'll do fine. One imperative: find yourself a Medical Home and establish a relationship with a primary care physician who welcomes the idea of working with you to improve and maintain your health. If you do nothing else, do this.

I recognize that many people who have the capacity to make the right choices still aren't going to, and here is where a trusting relationship with a primary care physician, or a health care team headed by a primary care physician, can be so valuable. Everyone needs a coach. Tiger Woods is the best golfer in the world, but even he has a coach. The truth about me is that I have a wife who sees to it that I eat correctly. In more ways than this, she has been my coach. I also recognize that there are folks who really don't have the capacity to make the right choices, and that we as a society have to help them. However, after a certain age, most of us know what's good for us in terms of our health and what isn't. The next step – that we then have to accept personal responsibility for those choices and their consequences – is where we look for a loophole, and our current health care system helps us out.

Because we as a society – for all the reasons I have set forth – have displaced individual <u>financial</u> responsibility for our health care onto our employers and the government, we also want to transfer our <u>personal</u> responsibility as well. This is moral hazard again. For example, I smoked a pipe for many years. I knew better – I'm a doctor – but I did it anyway. Now, on the day that I develop mouth cancer, is it your financial responsibility to help provide me with all kinds of expensive therapies? I don't think so, just as I don't think it's my responsibility to help you out financially when you reap the health consequences of all those gooey desserts. I'm not suggesting here that you should be able to dictate what I do or don't do; I'm saying that each of us should face the consequences – both financially and in terms of quality and length of life – of our individual lifestyle choices. Also, if and when you do become ill, you must be your own advocate – or be certain you have chosen an advocate ahead of time in case you are incapacitated. You cannot be passive, either before or during an illness.

As members of American society, you and I have a certain level of financial responsibility to each other when it comes to basic health care costs. This is the underlying principle of insurance – spread the risk and financial burden among many and it becomes tolerable for each person. At the same time, there does have to be a limit. Our society doesn't want to talk about that, for all the reasons I discussed in the previous chapter, but we're going to have to because we can no longer afford our current attitudes and behaviors.

One of the main reasons we don't have this kind of discussion is that most people don't fully realize that they're paying for their own health care, as well as the health care of others. As I've pointed out, whether it's through having your paycheck reduced by the amount your employer spends for health care insurance or the amount of taxes the government takes out to pay for various health care programs, you're paying. But because it's not something we can quantify – i.e., how many of your tax dollars go to pay for the financial consequences of my pipe smoking – the reality that you are paying for my behavior and I for yours somehow gets lost. We need to get that out in the open and then begin making some decisions about where and how to draw the line.

Another big reason we haven't had this kind of discussion is that when it comes to health care, nobody can tell you what anything really costs. Before we can humanely and accurately prioritize various types of treatment, we've got to know what they really cost. What's the true cost to a hospital for a given surgical procedure? What's the true cost to a drug company for developing and manufacturing a certain drug? What's the true cost to a medical device maker of developing and manufacturing an artificial knee? There are answers to these questions, but you're not going to get them from the companies themselves because they have a vested interest in keeping us ignorant. Pharmaceutical company CEOs will testify with a straight face that it cost $400 million to "develop" a new drug, knowing full well that half that was marketing, not research and development. I mentioned earlier that the four largest makers of artificial hips and knees paid $311 million to settle charges they paid kickbacks to surgeons who would use their products. Do you think they had to – and could afford to – pay kickbacks because their prices were fair and competitive?

To illustrate how backwards things have gotten, consider an example currently playing out in my home state of California, where health insurers are fighting vigorously against a law that would require them to pay out – gasp, oh the injustice of it all – at least 85% of the premiums they collect for patient care.

I mentioned earlier that the true role of an insurer should be as a repository and recycler of premiums, but the big insurers don't see it that way. According to the California Medical Association's 15th annual Knox-Keene Health Plan Expenditures Report, Blue Cross of California has spent less than 79% of premium dollars on patient care in fiscal year 2006-2007, with 17% going to profits and administration. This was the seventh year straight in which Blue Cross was below 80%.

It's called the Knox-Keene Health Plan Expenditures Report because of a California law called the Knox-Keene Act, which requires that no more than 15% of insurance company revenues go to administrative costs, including marketing. When the act became law, in 1975, the intent was to require insurers to spend 85% of collected premiums directly on medical care. For-profit health plans have since interpreted this to mean that their profits are an expense that can come from that 85%. In addition to Blue Cross, 11 other plans did not meet the 85% requirement for the 2006-2007 fiscal year covered by the report. Aetna Health Care, for example, spent only 81.4% of its premium dollars on patient care and Blue Shield just 82.1%.

Could these companies somehow manage to spend more on patients? It would seem so. For the same 2006-2007 time period, CIGNA HealthCare of California spent 94.3% on patients and Kaiser Foundation Health Plan 90.6%.

The effect of compelling insurers to return a minimum of 85% of premiums in the form of patient care would be enormous. In California alone, an additional $1 billion would be spent on patient care. Nationwide, of course, the gains would be much higher.

What's really astonishing – and outrageous – about this particular issue is not the percentages or dollar amounts involved, but that we have to have this fight at all. These are <u>our</u> premiums we're talking about. They don't "belong" to the insurance companies. Why should we be in the position of having to pry them back out of the insurers? If you pull back far enough to really think about it, the fact that California had to pass the Knox-Keene Act at all is off-the-charts absurd. That most of these same companies – more than 30 years later – are ignoring (violating) the law is even worse. It's a good example of how the health care industry has hijacked not just our money but our attitudes as well.

What all this really comes down to is the need for transparency. There's a saying regarding politics to the effect that sunlight is a great disinfectant. When people can really see what's going on, somehow those being observed behave more ethically. When people can see what things are really costing them, they are able to make more informed choices. This is what members of the medical industrial complex are fighting so vigorously, and here is where only we, the patients can do something about it.

The reality is that we must. Our health care system is collapsing around us. With some exceptions, the managers and top executives of publicly-held health care companies – the big pharmaceutical firms, the hospital chains, the medical device manufacturers, the insurance companies – are worrying about their quarterly earnings and stock options, not about you and me. Our politicians, at all levels, have been co-opted, as has medical academia. There's really nobody else left. We're it, and the time is right now.

I mentioned earlier that we each have more power than we believe. This is true in regard to our health care system because we are the source of its funding – through our taxes, the insurance premiums we pay and allow to be deducted from our paychecks, the checks we write for the co-pays, and all the other forms in which we spend our health care dollars. It's true also because millions of us are also shareholders in health care companies – through the stocks and mutual funds that we hold as individuals and in our company and union and personal pension plans. Again, this is our money, and we have a say in how and where it's invested.

It's time for each of us, to the extent that we can, to become advocates for health care that puts patients before profits. What that means in practice are actions like forming an employee group that goes to your HR department or union and asks to become part of the process by which your employer selects your health care plan, examining the stock holdings in your pension and/or retirement plan and asking the plan's investment manager to divest health care companies where pricing is not transparent, executive compensation is excessive, and the overall intent of management is to wring customers (that's us) dry. It means engaging in shareholder activism, i.e., attending the annual meetings of companies that comprise the medical-industrial complex and confronting the CEOs in a public forum about their values and behaviors, both as individuals and as corporate leaders. It means supporting patient advocacy groups (investigate them carefully first, some are fronts for special interests) with our time and money. It means speaking truth to power, which isn't easy but has to be done if we are to recapture control of health care.

Can't be done? Won't make any difference? Think back to the start of the environmental movement when scruffy-looking kids began badgering oil companies and other corporations about what they were doing to the earth. The early environmentalists were ridiculed, dismissed as radicals and fringe elements who really ought to get a bath and a job. Today, those same corporations are scrambling to "out-green" each other. Some of it is window-dressing, of course, but there's also been a real change in the way corporations think and act when it comes to the environment. And despite what their ads may say now, those corporations didn't change their ways because they were worried about the air and sea and earth, they changed because they were worried about the effects that environmental activism was having on customer loyalty, shareholder support, their own employees, legislative policies, and, ultimately, their very viability as publicly-held companies. Sustained pressure by customers and shareholders can have a very real effect on the behavior of public companies, and this is even truer today than it was in the infancy of the environmental movement. A key point: Don't wait until you're sick or injured to act on this. By then, you are both personally vulnerable and pre-occupied with getting better. Do something now!

At this point, we come to a central question: What is the proper role of the publicly-held, for-profit health care company? Is it above all to maximize profits for the benefit of shareholders? Many people would say yes, that social goals are the province of government, charitable foundations and private individuals. They would argue further that the taxes corporations pay can be directed via government policies towards furthering those social objectives the public approves at the ballot-box. Asking corporations to do anything except maximize profits is distorting their function, this group would say, and their view has dominated for quite some time. Certainly, deregulation, laissez-faire and the "will of the marketplace" have been the prevailing principles when it comes to business for several decades.

What has adherence to these "principles" brought us? How well have they served us? Our finance, housing, manufacturing and auto industries, to pick just a few, are in shambles. We are beholden to other nations, many of whom despise us, for the oil and capital our economy must have to function. Our national debt, most of it held by foreign entities, has swollen enormously. Our currency has lost a significant amount of value. I could go on, but you can fill in other areas where we've lost ground yourself. The point is: Can anyone seriously contend that what Big Business has been doing is working for us as a nation or as individuals?

Macro-economics is not the focus of this book, and I do not wish to stray too far afield. However, I think it is high time for us to rethink how we regard – and yes, regulate – companies that supply the necessities of life – food, shelter, transportation, energy, and my area of expertise, health care. This is particularly true because health care is not a free market. You can trade down (or up) on the car you drive, the house you live in and what you have for dinner, but when you need an appendectomy, there's no bargaining. In those circumstances, is maximizing profits the proper role of the health care company? Again, don't lose sight of where those profits come from – they come from you and me.

Eventually, this becomes a question of values. If we are to find our way to a new era in health care, one that puts patients before profits but also recognizes that companies must make money in order to survive and innovate, we're going to have to reflect on, discuss, and ultimately decide what our values are in this regard. This is a major reason why transparency on the part of health care companies – on prices, on how much is spent on true research and development and how much on marketing, on executive compensation, on the effect of stock options, and in other key areas – is so important. We can't really evaluate most health care companies and determine what they're really doing (as opposed to what they say they're doing), because there's no transparency. And don't think for a moment that health care CEOs don't realize this. They rely on it.

So more transparency is one of the things we must push hard for. But assuming for a moment that we are able to view all the participants in the health care equation – patients, providers and payers, broadly speaking – more clearly, how should we evaluate them? What are our values when it comes to health care?

We all play significant roles in the health care. Patients who neglect their individual health and then expect providers to do whatever it takes to deal with the consequences are placing a burden on everyone else. Providers – individual and corporate – who try to make health care a road to riches are exploiting their fellow man, pure and simple. Payers who manipulate the intricacies of our health care system to maximize their profits and pump up their stock prices are doing the same.

Judging blatantly selfish acts such as these is straightforward. More difficult to arrive at – and even more difficult to put into practice – is the inverse, not what health care participants shouldn't be doing but what they should. Here I would suggest that the process begins in the mirror. What do each of us as individuals believe in, and are we walking the walk? Do we believe in a "me" society or a "we" society?

We each have to have this "conversation" with ourselves because if we don't know what we believe in as individuals, we can't know what our values are when it comes to health care. That means we can't know what standards to apply to ourselves as patients, and to providers and payers. For example, if you really believe that life is about taking care of Number One, then you should love our current health care system, because that's what it's about too.

As I've suggested earlier, one of the reasons and perhaps even the primary reason that our health care system got hijacked was because we don't know what we believe in anymore. We are always on quicksand – lurching from one position to another based on spin and slickness – rather than making decisions and choices based on a firm, philosophical footing. If I know what my values are and what I should be doing, then I have a foundation from which to push those values upwards – to my family, my community, my profession, my state, my nation. I can think critically about what politicians are espousing, what my friends and colleagues are doing, and about the questions involving not just health care but other issues as well.

I've laid out some of the things I believe in regarding health care. I believe a basic level of affordable health care is a need, not a want, and should be available to all. I believe everyone should take an active role in maintaining their health. I believe that physicians and other providers, including corporations, should be motivated primarily by a desire to help others, not the urge to get rich. I believe payers should function as repositories and recyclers of the money they collect, nothing more. Most of all, I believe the doctor-patient relationship is the cornerstone of health care and should be re-elevated to its rightful place.

I could go on, but the real point is not what I believe but what you believe and what you're doing about it. I don't believe in a single-payer system because I think it represents the ultimate displacement of responsibility, but if you do, go for it. The same goes for other issues. Sit down and figure out what you believe in regarding health care. Discuss your beliefs with others – there are clubs over the country that meet monthly to talk about the latest hot book, how about starting a club in your neighborhood to discuss what to do about health care? When you reach consensus on some issues, take the next step and begin to push for change – at your employer, from your elected officials, from the health care companies, and from yourself. Write letters to the editor, get petitions going, start a blog, enlist others in the cause, put your creativity to work.

This may sound vague, and if you were expecting a four-point program that would magically solve our health care problems, I have news for you. There are no silver bullets or free-lunch solutions. Real change, lasting change is only going to occur as the result of a grassroots movement that pushes ethics and values up into our health care system. It's got to be bottom-up, because what we have now is top-down and I think you know how well it's working. Do something about it!

Chapter Twelve

THE FUTURE OF AMERICAN HEALTH CARE

What Will Happen if We Don't Take Responsibility for our Health and Health Care System; What Can Happen if We Do

As I mentioned at the beginning of this book, one of the few positive signs in our current health care crisis is that no one can credibly argue that what we're doing is working – for anyone. Although they have different ideas on how to fix things, patients, providers and payers are all fed up with what's going on. Even so, I don't think that most people fully understand how serious and pervasive a mess we have created in health care. The reason is that our so-called system is still limping along. The overall quality, accessibility, cost-effectiveness and humanity of American health care is declining, but we haven't had – and aren't going to have – a single, dramatic wakeup call along the line of 9/11. Instead, as hospitals and emergency rooms continue to close, doctors leave the profession, costs and insurance premiums rise, and we focus increasingly on episodic, disease oriented-care at the expense of prevention and wellness, our health care system is slowly seizing up. This is happening even though we are spending more and more on health care every year. This situation, even if it was producing decent health care for Americans, is obviously unsustainable.

In circumstances like this, where people know things can't go on like they are but don't know what to do about it, there's a tendency to reach for simplistic solutions and convenient scapegoats. This is what's behind the trial balloons praising single-payer systems (government-run health care). Single-payer systems don't work, because they are the ultimate abdication of personal responsibility, and as such, cannot produce quality health care on an individual level. I don't want to engage here in a long discussion on this issue, so I'll reduce it to an apt slogan: If you like dealing with the DMV, you'll love single-payer health care.

On the opposite side of the political spectrum from single-payer advocates are those who contend that "the market" should be allowed to function freely in regard to health care. I think it's fairly apparent that health care is not a free market simply because people don't choose to contract cancer or get hit by cars, but there's another problem with this school of thought, one that has become unmistakable as the first decade of the 21st Century heads for the finish line. We are experiencing another Depression – let's be honest – and the roots of it lie in the bottomless greed of those on Wall Street and in corporate boardrooms who cast aside ethics and morals and common decency in the pursuit of more money than they could possibly spend. For God's sake, what do you do with a $20 million bonus when you already have $100 million? How can someone repeatedly dupe regulators and swindle investors year after year after year until the tab hits $50 billion?

This is where unregulated free markets eventually but inevitably take you – in this case, millions of people losing their homes, jobs, and life savings because of the unchecked avarice of a relative few. In terms of health care, free markets provide an environment in which CEOs of non-profit hospitals can leverage the compensation of their for-profit colleagues so as to earn almost $500,000 a year at the same time as exorbitant medical costs force millions of people – the very folks nonprofits are supposed to be treating – into personal bankruptcies. It's the obscene spectacle of Big Pharma buying research findings that favor their products, medical device manufacturers paying kickbacks to physicians, hospitals charging $6 for an aspirin, insurance companies reneging when their customers have the nerve to actually file claims, and pensioners having to choose between their meds and dinner. Welcome to the jungle.

Like most polarizing issues, there are zealots on both side of this one. Single-payer advocates try to brand their opponents as rapacious capitalists and free market proponents label their adversaries as socialists. Neither charge is true, and all the inflammatory rhetoric makes reforming our health care system very difficult to achieve. But reform we must. If our country could somehow have flashed forward from what we had when I entered medical school to the circumstances we find ourselves in today, I don't think anyone would have started down the path. Things have to change.

What I have tried to show in this book is that we went astray starting with the government's intrusion into health care via Medicare and Medicaid. While presumably well-intentioned, this attempt to insulate people cradle-to-grave from the realities of life – including the fact that we all eventually get ill and die – opened the door to all manner of mischief perpetrated by so-called "market forces." Although the road was circuitous, it was this original error that ultimately led to the mess we're in today. We shouldn't make that mistake again.

It's not my intent to re-fight the battles of the '60s. We're not going back to where we were then, and wherever we are going with regard to health care, we have to start from where we are now. We're not going to revolutionize American health care – we have to "evolutionize" it. This is the key point that people all along the political spectrum need to understand and accept. We have to work with what we have – we're not going to drive either government or capitalism completely out of health care, nor should we want to. There has to be some baseline level of health care available to all regardless of income, because we can hardly do less in a civilized society, and government is the appropriate entity to finance and facilitate this, although not to dictate how that care is delivered. At the same time, the private sector has a role in health care too. Innovation, efficiency, customer (patient) satisfaction – these are not hallmarks of government. There's also a place for the profit motive – when true entrepreneurs, individual or corporate, invent or develop something that advances medicine and benefits patients, those entrepreneurs should reap a reward.

So if we want both government and the private sector to have a role in health care, but at the same time we don't want either party running the show completely, to whom do we turn? There's really only one answer, which is why I chose it as the title of this book: We the Patients. This is the single role that binds us all together. We have to re-assert control of our health care system, and of our individual health, while at the same time acknowledging that in today's world, what we do, the choices we make, have a significant impact on others.

One of the reasons, perhaps the primary reason, that our society, our economy and our health care system are in such dire straits is that somewhere along the way we stopped caring about each other and started worrying only about Number One. What we are seeing play out in the economy is a prime example. People who knew at heart that they couldn't afford the houses they wanted bought them anyway, aided and abetted by loan officers who cared only about their commissions. Houses came to be seen not as places to raise a family but as ways to turn a quick buck. Absurd loans were packaged into exotic mortgage-backed securities by financiers who cared only about the embedded profits, blessed by rating agencies that knew better but wanted the business, and sold off to banks and other institutions whose executives were focused exclusively on their own bonuses and stock options. At every step along the way, the individuals involved worried only about their own slice of the pie and how they could maximize it. This includes politicians who pushed social policies that helped put people into houses they couldn't afford. Nobody was willing to be accountable – and they still aren't. Everyone is lining up at the government trough, not just asking but expecting to be bailed out, regardless of both the fact that they largely got themselves into trouble and that the long-term consequences of rescuing them will fall largely on others.

The dynamics are essentially the same in health care. We've abandoned individual responsibility in favor of a "me-first" attitude that somehow assumes people are entitled not only to unlimited medical care but actually to enjoy robust health without bothering to practice the lifestyle habits that produce it. We want good health and good health care, but we feel that someone else – insurance companies, our employers and the government – should foot the bill. And all along the way are those who aid and abet. TV commercials promise us vigor in a pill, politicians tell us that heretofore undiscovered "efficiencies" will pay for costly new initiatives, and CEOs of insurance, hospital, and pharmaceutical companies claim that their excessive profits and absurd salaries are justified because of the incredible complexity of today's health care system. Meanwhile, what really matters – a patient and physician having an honest, face-to-face dialogue about a problem and how to treat it – has been replaced by the 10-minute appointment, a scribbled prescription and referral to a specialist who sees the patient as a kidney or lung or heart instead of a person. This is what we've come to, and it is unraveling just like the financial house of cards that has collapsed on our heads.

Remember the crazed anchorman in the movie "Network" who urged viewers to go to their windows, fling them open and shout, "I'm as mad as hell and I'm not going to take it anymore"? Well, he had a point. Nothing is going to really change until each of us decides that we've had enough and that we're not going to take it anymore. That doesn't mean turning to Washington to solve the problem, because that's essentially what led us into this mess in the first place. It means acknowledging each of us has to be responsible for our individual health and, collectively, for our health care system.

Those who pass themselves off as experts on our health care system are forever reminding us that all the issues and mechanisms and tradeoffs involved in changing the system are incredibly complex. These observations are usually self-serving, and they also overlook a critically important point. Our health care system is complex because we have made it so, not because it has to be that way. As I have discussed, we never laid down a blueprint for what we wanted and then followed those specifications in constructing our system. Instead, we took what was an imperfect but essentially functional way of delivering health care and tinkered with it over and over and over again. It wasn't really broken, but it sure is now. We have allowed government to decide too many things, let greed elbow aside ethical business practices, and forsaken our individual responsibilities in favor of adolescent, something-for-nothing fantasies.

This is not a political book, and I don't want to get into a partisan debate over the role of government in health care except to say that 40-plus years in medicine have convinced me that it should involve general principles rather than detailed regulations. Rule books compiled by bureaucrats almost always stifle initiative and innovation while simultaneously daring those who would game the system for profit to find a loophole. Where government can be useful is in broadly defining what minimum level of health care should be available to all regardless of their ability to pay. This might include such things as childhood immunizations, basic diagnostic tests such as pap smears and cholesterol screening, and educational initiatives that stress good nutrition and daily aerobic exercise. Where government should not get involved in health care is in the specifics of what constitutes appropriate treatment, which is a matter to be discussed and decided between doctor and patient, or in the details of how a medical practice or hospital or clinic operates.

If we really want to improve our health care system – and our collective health – we have to do something fundamentally different, not apply another patch in the form of another government program. There is no silver bullet or "techno-fix" – we have to rethink the health care system from top to bottom.

The national health care model we have today, for the reasons I have discussed, is based essentially on providing high-cost healthcare services to people with chronic conditions. We are disease-oriented and reactive – we wait until people are really in trouble and then throw money at their problems. Because of this, three out of every four health care dollars we spend go to treat chronic illnesses such as asthma, diabetes, heart disease, and others.

Although genetics and luck play a role, most chronic disease is essentially lifestyle-related. How we live, individually and collectively, determines in large part how and when we die. Plunk yourself down on the couch every night with a Big Mac and a six-pack and you're virtually certain to have a most unpleasant last few years of life that are also quite expensive for the rest of us. Placate your children with video games and sugary sodas instead of making them (yes, making) get out and walk and bike and move and you're setting them on a road that generally ends quite badly. As an aside, we need to get PE back in the schools.

Unfortunately, more and more Americans are making self-destructive choices. About 15% of us were obese in the mid-1990s. Now it's about 25%, and this increase has occurred in a little more than a decade. The obesity picture for children is nothing short of horrible – the adolescent obesity rate is up threefold from 20 years ago. Since obesity is a primary cause of chronic conditions like heart disease and diabetes, we're creating a new generation that is predisposed to the same chronic illnesses that are already consuming the majority of our health care dollars and making the final years of millions of Americans miserable indeed.

Why are we allowing this to happen? I believe a large part of it is that we don't personally feel the financial pain that our lifestyle decisions – and those of others – create. Only 13% of the total dollars being spent on health care actually come directly out of consumers' pockets. There's this illusion that somebody else (government, employers, insurance companies) is paying and, even worse, that we're entitled to have somebody else pay. One of the reasons people obey speeding laws is that tickets are expensive and they drive your insurance rates up. There is no similar incentive in health care (unless you want to count health insurers who cancel your policy if you file a claim). Your doctor can urge you to do this or that, but nothing happens (immediately) if you don't obey the rules of a healthy lifestyle.

As many studies have demonstrated, when people have to pay out of pocket for their health care, they make different choices. Those choices aren't always the right ones, but the fact that the individual has skin in the game changes the decision-making. Again, this is a major reason why government-run health care systems don't work – responsibility is shifted away from the individual. It's also the rationale behind Health Savings Accounts, which while not perfect, do put more responsibility onto the individual patient.

I mentioned earlier that many so-called "experts" spend a lot of time proclaiming how complex our health care problems are, with the underlying implication being that we need such experts to help us solve them. Actually, our core problem is pretty straightforward. At all levels – individual patient, family, employer, provider, insurer, industry, government, etc. – we're not taking responsibility for our actions and we're not holding others accountable for theirs. Individuals who smoke or overeat are placing a burden on all of us, as are families who let their kids zombie-out in front of their computers, doctors who prescribe instead of counsel, HMO executives who worship profits – you can make your own list. Until and unless this changes, our health care system will continue to deteriorate. In other words, we have to change individual behavior.

This next point can be portrayed as cold-hearted, but it's not, it's simply realistic. While I'm not suggesting in any way that we abandon them, fundamental long-term reform of our health care system means focusing not on those who are already ill but on those who are not. The way we operate now – wait until people get sick, very frequently as a result of their own lifestyle choices, and then spend huge sums of money on their health issues – means that about 10% of our population drives roughly 70% of our healthcare expenditures and policy priorities. That's simply not sustainable, especially since our population is aging. We can't fix this problem by focusing on the manifestation – we have to work on the cause.

What this means, in broad terms, is that we need to change how we think about health care in a number of critical areas. We need to focus on long-term initiatives in the areas of education, wellness and prevention, and this should begin in the home and continue in the doctor-patient relationship – the medical home. Layered on top of this, we need a system of incentives that reward and reinforce positive lifestyle choices and inhibit negative ones. This is tricky territory, but we have to go there. Entrenched behaviors don't change spontaneously – we have to give them a nudge. The best place for this to happen is in the family, which is where values and behaviors are learned, or should be.

One of the most unfortunate aspects of the times we're living in is that the role and importance of the family has somehow been devalued. Why this has happened is an enormous topic by itself, and outside the parameters of this book, but I don't think there can be any argument that it has happened. Although it may offend some feminists, I'll go further and say that we have also devalued the role and importance of motherhood. I believe very strongly that women are equal, should have professional careers if they want them, and should be paid the same as a man for doing the same work. But while holding those beliefs, I also respect and honor the roles of homemaker, counselor, nurturer and all the other critically important aspects of motherhood. Our society seems to have lost sight of the fact that being a good mother is a difficult, demanding, full-time occupation, and we're seeing the consequences in many areas, one of them being health care. If we want people to make better choices about their individual health, that has to be learned in the home. If we want people to be responsible and accountable and concerned about others, those qualities have to be instilled in the home.

At the same time, since health insurance is still job-based for most Americans, we may also need for employers to be more proactive in terms of lifestyle behaviors. For example, should an employee who refuses to stop smoking be eligible for the same company-wide health care premiums as those who don't smoke? What about an employee who is grossly obese, or alcoholic? The assertion that these people are only hurting themselves simply isn't true. They are hurting their loved ones, and when they drive up the insurance premiums of their fellow employees, they are hurting them as well.

I understand that this is more complicated than just saying that people "choose" to smoke, or overeat, or drink too much. I also recognize that there are all sorts of other implications to these questions, not to mention various "civil rights" groups eager to litigate. However, the reality is that we need to start thinking – and acting – differently if we want real change in health care.

While we're focusing on prevention and wellness among those who are still healthy, we also have to care for those who are already ill. We have a moral obligation to care for them and we should do this by recognizing the primary role of the doctor-patient relationship, by empowering physicians, by continuing to invest in new technologies and medications, by recognizing that diseases of the elderly are going to become more and more prominent, and by extending the empathy and compassion that all of us will want when our time comes. But this means, among other things, recognizing that life ends. Again, I'm not suggesting in any way that we write off those who have chronic illnesses, only that we recognize that we can't outspend and out-treat diseases caused primarily by lifestyle choices.

I have discussed the problems in our health care system in some detail because just as a doctor must identify an illness in order to treat it, I believe we cannot address these problems unless we know what they really are and where they originated. But I also want to offer a vision of what we can gain by thinking about our individual health and our health care system in a different way, and by acting on that new way of thinking. Here I will quote Einstein: "We can't solve problems by using the same kind of thinking we used when we created them." So let's discard the "let's apply another patch" mentality that has dominated the health care discussion in favor of a bigger picture, one that hopefully can motivate us all to think and act differently.

I believe that the great majority of Americans can live longer and more satisfying lives, enjoy good health in their later years and face the inevitability of death with serenity and acceptance. All these things are within our individual and collective grasp, right here, right now. They are affordable and available, simply by turning away from what we have been conditioned to believe and instead recognizing certain natural realities and living in ways that respect our own individual health and the fact that our personal choices affect society as a whole.

I have attempted in this book to sketch out what happened to American health care over the last 40-plus years and what that has meant to us on an individual basis. One of the themes I hope has come through loud and clear is that we have been repeatedly manipulated by groups that do not have our best interests at heart. This includes the giant, publicly-held hospital, insurance, and pharmaceutical companies, medical schools, our legislators, government bureaucracies, and, it grieves me to acknowledge, some physicians and physicians groups as well. Simply put, your institutions aren't looking out for you.

At the same time, no amount of lobbying, advertising, back-room politicking or Wall Street chicanery can obliterate some very positive realities regarding our individual and collective health. For example, good, nutritious food is widely available in this country. It may take longer to obtain and prepare, but it's accessible. Exercise that makes a big difference in individual health – walking, biking, swimming, yoga etc. – requires only that we get out and do it. Spiritual development, more quality time with family and friends – almost all of the things that really matter in life are there to be experienced and enjoyed. We don't need another pill, or test, or syndrome, or government program to take advantage of these things – and generally speaking they will do more to keep you healthy than anything else. But we can't look elsewhere in adopting these values and behaviors. We have to acknowledge that how we live – meaning the dozens of seemingly small choices we make every day – affects our current health, the kind of death we're likely to have, and the positive or negative effect we're having on society as a whole.

It's always useful, and especially so when in the midst of a thorny problem, to invert – to think about what would happen if you did the opposite of what you've been doing. What would happen if I really did get out and walk 30 minutes every day, no matter what? What would happen if I stopped blaming my (spouse, employer, neighbor – fill in the blank) for the problems that exists between us? What would happen if I told my kids they could only watch two hours of TV a day? And – here's the punchline – instead of going to the doctor only when I was sick, what would happen if instead I went while I was well and asked, "How can I stay healthy?"

Although we've been conditioned to regard it as something we turn to only when something is wrong, health care can and should be a great ally in our lives. Medicine has advanced enormously in recent years and even greater leaps are possible in the years ahead, especially if we re-focus research away from what will make the most money for Big Pharma and onto what will do the greatest good for the greatest number of people. The tools we need to enjoy healthier lives are here, and more are coming. We need only to pick them up and use them. Many people already have – the anecdotal evidence is all around us in the form of people who are living healthy, productive, joyous lives well into their older years. Although some of us are dealt tough hands genetically, your chances of living well and living long are better than they have ever been – if you take responsibility for your own health.

As part of this, we also have to take responsibility for our own death. People shy away from this topic, but the acceptance of death helps give meaning to life. We experience this anecdotally every so often when someone famous, or perhaps someone close to us, dies at an early age. We reflect, albeit briefly, on how we are spending our time, how we are living our lives, what our priorities are. All too often, those thoughts are then swept aside by the next immediate problem and their power to effect personal change is lost to us. Without being melancholy or maudlin, I want to suggest that instead we stay with those thoughts long enough to let them guide us in how we are living today.

Because I have spent my life in medicine, I have seen many people die. Consequently, I am acutely aware that there are good deaths and bad deaths, some extremely bad. And while many factors – luck and genetics among them – play a role in the specifics of the destination we all share, I have seen many people spend their final days with dignity and grace. Almost without exception, they were people who took personal responsibility for their health early on and recognized that there were no shortcuts or loopholes in that equation. Almost without exception, they were people who did not deny the reality of death but used it instead as a way of examining how they lived their lives. Accepting that life is finite – for ourselves and for others – provides powerful motivation to live meaningful lives, to love and be loved, to further causes greater than our own self-interest and the quick buck.

Death is not an enemy to be avoided and denied. In fact, it is an ally, a reminder that life is too brief and too precious to be squandered on things that ultimately don't matter. Let me put it this way: If you knew you were going to die 24 hours from now, who would you call, what would you say, how and with whom would you spend tonight and tomorrow morning? Now let me ask the real question: What are you waiting for?

The ripple effects from the personal acceptance of life's realities and responsibilities are enormous, perhaps almost incomprehensible in today's "it's somebody else's fault" society. People can exchange a depressive defeated existence for an exhilarating sense of personal empowerment and the realization that almost anything worthwhile is within our grasp if we are willing to do what's required. We don't have to be sick and tired and helpless and end our days tethered to machines that prolong what is by then a miserable existence. But we can't delegate or abdicate our personal responsibility in matters concerning our own health.

We are experiencing what amounts to a giant wake-up call in this country. Our societal institutions have failed us, pure and simple, and we need to rethink them from top to bottom. At the individual level, personal responsibility has taken a back seat to immediate gratification, with devastating consequences. It's time for personal responsibility and accountability to make a comeback – and again, this has to start in the home, with the family. If a person doesn't have these values when they leave the nest, they're highly unlikely to develop them. We have to start at the source, not downstream.

While we may have very different ideas on how things should change on a macro level, when it comes to our individual health and, by extension, our health care system, things seem pretty clear. We need to teach and practice wellness and prevention. We need to be accountable to ourselves, to those we love, and to our society as a whole, for the lifestyle choices we make every day. We need to confront all those who are exploiting patients for the sake of profits. We need to be examples instead of excuses, and it all has to start with the person in the mirror. If this book contributes to a rebirth of those values and behaviors, I'll give the man in my mirror a smile.

Thank you for reading my book. If it made sense to you, please adopt some of the suggestions and pass this book on to someone you care about.

ABOUT THE AUTHOR

Sam JW Romeo became a board-certified Family Physician in 1970 and went on to a distinguished career in medicine that has taken him all over the United States. He worked in rural emergency rooms, served as President of the Idaho Academy of Family Physicians, President of the Accreditation Association for Ambulatory Health Care, Inc. (AAAHC), and was senior associate dean at the Saint Louis University School of Medicine, Medical College of Wisconsin and University of Southern California School of Medicine. He founded and was CEO of the nation's first fully-accredited Independent Physician's Association, a medical group of 2,500 physicians associated with the USC School of Medicine. He did his residency in the Medical Corps of the U.S. Navy, where he rose to the rank of Commander.

Measuring and improving the quality of health care has been a foremost concern of Dr. Romeo's throughout his career, and he has chaired the Performance

Measurement Initiative of the AAAHC's Institute for Quality Improvement. He recently chaired an AAAHC task force developing standards for what is now being called the Medical Home, an important subject in his book.

Dr. Romeo, who obtained his MBA while working as a physician, also understands health care from a business perspective. He held positions as CEO of small HMOs and as Medical Director for a Fortune 1000 corporation. He is a Fellow of the American College of Physician Executives, and in 1998 was named Physician Executive of the Year by the American College of Medical Practice Executives.

Dr. Romeo and his wife Patty have passed on the love of medicine to their six children, with five becoming physicians and the sixth a Licensed Clinical Social Worker. He co-founded and is currently President and CEO of the Tower Health and Wellness Center in Turlock, California, and Medical Director of the Tower Surgery Center. In his infrequent spare time, he can often be found at events involving one or more of 21 grandchildren, or making furniture for their bedrooms.

For more information, please visit www.wethepatients.org.

www.ingramcontent.com/pod-product-compliance
Lightning Source LLC
Chambersburg PA
CBHW071414170526
45165CB00001B/274